■ DRUGS
The Straight Facts

Sleep Aids

DRUGS The Straight Facts

Alcohol

Antidepressants

Body Enhancement Products

Cocaine

Date Rape Drugs

Designer Drugs

Diet Pills

Ecstasy

Hallucinogens

Heroin

Inhalants

Marijuana

Nicotine

Prescription Pain Relievers

Ritalin and Other Methylphenidate-Containing Drugs

Sleep Aids

■ DRUGS
The Straight Facts

Sleep Aids

M. Foster Olive

Consulting Editor
David J. Triggle
University Professor
School of Pharmacy and Pharmaceutical Sciences
State University of New York at Buffalo

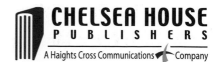

CHELSEA HOUSE
PUBLISHERS
A Haights Cross Communications Company
Philadelphia

CHELSEA HOUSE PUBLISHERS
VP, NEW PRODUCT DEVELOPMENT Sally Cheney
DIRECTOR OF PRODUCTION Kim Shinners
CREATIVE MANAGER Takeshi Takahashi
MANUFACTURING MANAGER Diann Grasse

Staff for SLEEP AIDS
SENIOR EDITOR Melissa Williams
ASSOCIATE EDITOR Beth Reger
PRODUCTION EDITOR Bonnie Cohen
PHOTO EDITOR Sarah Bloom
SERIES & COVER DESIGNER Terry Mallon
LAYOUT 21st Century Publishing and Communications, Inc.

A Haights Cross Communications ⌖ Company

http://www.chelseahouse.com

First Printing

1 3 5 7 9 8 6 4 2

Library of Congress Cataloging-in-Publication Data

Olive, M. Foster.
    Sleep aids/M. Foster Olive.
        p. cm.—(Drugs, the straight facts)
    Includes bibliographical references and index.
    ISBN 0-7910-8200-8
1. Hypnotics. 2. Sleep. I. Title. II. Series.
RM325.O45 2006
615'.782—dc22

                                                                2005016612

Table of Contents

The Use and Abuse of Drugs

The issues associated with drug use and abuse in contemporary society are vexing subjects, fraught with political agendas and ideals that often obscure essential information that teens need to know to have intelligent discussions about how to best deal with the problems associated with drug use and abuse. *Drugs: The Straight Facts* aims to provide this essential information through straightforward explanations of how an individual drug or group of drugs works in both therapeutic and non-therapeutic conditions; with historical information about the use and abuse of specific drugs; with discussion of drug policies in the United States; and with an ample list of further reading.

From the start, the series uses the word *"drug"* to describe psychoactive substances that are used for medicinal or non-medicinal purposes. Included in this broad category are substances that are legal or illegal. It is worth noting that humans have used many of these substances for hundreds, if not thousands of years. For example, traces of marijuana and cocaine have been found in Egyptian mummies; the use of peyote and Amanita fungi has long been a component of religious ceremonies worldwide; and alcohol production and consumption have been an integral part of many human cultures' social and religious ceremonies. One can speculate about why early human societies chose to use such drugs. Perhaps, anything that could provide relief from the harshness of life—anything that could make the poor conditions and fatigue associated with hard work easier to bear—was considered a welcome tonic. Life was likely to be, according to the seventeenth century English philosopher Thomas Hobbes, *"poor, nasty, brutish and short."* One can also speculate about modern human societies' continued use and abuse of drugs. Whatever the reasons, the consequences of sustained drug use are not insignificant—addiction, overdose, incarceration, and drug wars—and must be dealt with by an informed citizenry.

The problem that faces our society today is how to break

the connection between our demand for drugs and the willingness of largely outside countries to supply this highly profitable trade. This is the same problem we have faced since narcotics and cocaine were outlawed by the Harrison Narcotic Act of 1914, and we have yet to defeat it despite current expenditures of approximately $20 billion per year on "the war on drugs." The first step in meeting any challenge is always an intelligent and informed citizenry. The purpose of this series is to educate our readers so that they can make informed decisions about issues related to drugs and drug abuse.

SUGGESTED ADDITIONAL READING

David T. Courtwright, *Forces of Habit. Drugs and the Making of the Modern World.* Cambridge, Mass.: Harvard University Press, 2001. David Courtwright is Professor of History at the University of North Florida.

Richard Davenport-Hines, *The Pursuit of Oblivion. A Global History of Narcotics.* New York: Norton, 2002. The author is a professional historian and a member of the Royal Historical Society.

Aldous Huxley, *Brave New World.* New York: Harper & Row, 1932. Huxley's book, written in 1932, paints a picture of a cloned society devoted only to the pursuit of happiness.

David J. Triggle, Ph.D.
University Professor
School of Pharmacy and Pharmaceutical Sciences
State University of New York at Buffalo

1

What Is This Thing We Call "Sleep?"

"There is a time for many words, and there is also a time for sleep."

—Homer, *The Odyssey*

It's 8:00 P.M. and you have a huge test tomorrow that determines half of your grade in chemistry class. You haven't studied nearly enough and you figure you need at least six more hours to cover all the material. So, you have a cola or a cup of coffee and stay up late to finish studying. Then 11:00 P.M. rolls around and your mind starts to drift and you think about other things. At 1:00 A.M., you feel your eyelids getting heavy, so you turn on some music to try and stay awake. As you keep reading from your textbook, your mind drifts further and you find yourself listening to the music more than paying attention to reading. By 2:00 A.M., none of the chemistry reading is sinking in and you decide you'll just have to wake up early to finish studying. You set your alarm for 6:00 A.M. and, as your head hits the pillow, you start to think about the test and how much it means for your grade. Suddenly, the tiredness is gone and your mind races with worry. You toss and turn for an hour before you finally drift off to sleep.

The alarm goes off at 6:00 A.M. and you barely manage to wake up enough to hit the snooze bar. Fifteen minutes later, it goes off again, and again you hit the snooze bar. You repeat this process until suddenly, at 7:00 A.M., you wake with panic as you realize you never finished studying and you're going to be late for school and the test, which happens to be your first-period class. After a rushed breakfast and a shower, you throw on some clothes and dash out the door to school, arriving just seconds before the first-period bell rings. The teacher places the test in front of you, and all you can think is, "Sleep, that cursed sleep! I could have aced this exam if it weren't for sleep!"

Sleep: sometimes it seems like a huge thorn in our sides and such a waste of time. It gets in the way of our studying, socializing, and other fun activities like Internet surfing and watching late night movies. Yet, at other times, when we are dog-tired after a long day at school, sleep feels as good as a jump in the pool on a hot summer's day. Whether we like it or not, sleep is inevitable—we all must sleep, no matter how hard or long we try to fight it. Even birds, other mammals, fish, and insects—most living things—sleep or rest in some way or another. And it's not just a short nap we need: humans actually spend approximately one-third of our lives (8 out of every 24 hours) sleeping.

WHAT IS SLEEP?

Historically, sleep has been considered a time of mere inactivity for the mind and body to rejuvenate itself. Some philosophers have even considered it a complete waste of time. However, 20th century scientific and medical research into the phenomenon of sleep has revealed that these simplistic views of sleep are not at all accurate. Human and animal sleep is actually a complex series of different states of consciousness orchestrated by the brain. Sleep is essential for our health and well-being. For the purposes of this chapter, we will focus on human sleep. However, there are some fascinating facts about sleep in other animals: see the box on page 15 for more details.

Sleep typically consists of two main phases—**rapid eye movement (REM) sleep** (sometimes called "active sleep") and **non-REM sleep** (also called "quiet sleep"). Non-REM sleep can be further divided into different stages. For example, when a person first falls asleep, he or she enters what is called Stage 1 non-REM sleep, when the mind "drifts" into random thought patterns accompanied by the relaxing of muscles and the occasional "twitch" of the arms or legs. Next, the person advances through Stages 2, 3, and 4 of non-REM sleep, which are progressively deeper, more physically restorative stages of sleep.

After about 60 to 90 minutes of non-REM sleep, the body enters REM sleep (Figure 1.1). This stage of sleep is like no other state of consciousness and is when most dreaming occurs. REM sleep is so-named because it is characterized by rapid movements of the eyes back and forth (behind closed eyelids, usually). In addition, breathing and heart rate patterns become irregular and more rapid. Also, a complete loss of all skeletal muscle tone is experienced (i.e., your arms, legs, neck, back, and facial muscles are completely limp and you are, in a sense, temporarily paralyzed). This loss of muscle tone is called **atonia**, and without it you would actually act out whatever it is you are doing in your dreams. This happens in people with a rare sleep disorder called *REM without atonia* or *REM behavior disorder* (see Chapter 2). Although the skeletal muscles are inactive during REM sleep, brain scans of people during their sleep have revealed that the brain is extremely active during REM sleep (Figure 1.2), and at times more active than it is when you are awake! (Animals dream, too. Have you ever seen a dog or cat look like it is trying to run when it is dreaming?)

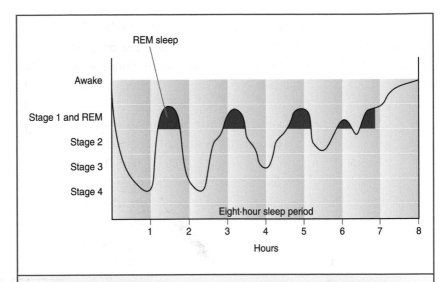

Figure 1.1 In a typical night's sleep, the brain cycles through REM sleep and the various stages of non-REM sleep many times. After the first 60–90 minutes of the various stages of non-REM sleep, the first REM period occurs and lasts about 10–30 minutes, and then the person falls back into non-REM sleep. These cycles of REM and non-REM sleep repeat several times during the night. As the night goes on, periods of REM sleep become longer in duration and more frequent. It is thought that dreams are more likely to be remembered when the person is awakened from REM as opposed to non-REM sleep. Thus, the likelihood of remembering your dreams is much greater in the morning, when you are spending most of your time in REM sleep, than in the middle of the night when fewer REM episodes have occurred and are more interspersed with non-REM sleep.

SLEEP IS A BIOLOGICAL RHYTHM

Most humans sleep at night when it is dark (this is called being *diurnal*, or active during the day), although some people with jobs that make them work through the night must adapt to sleep during the day. But many species of animals, such as rats, mice, and raccoons, are *nocturnal*, or active at night. Whether we sleep during the night or day, our sleep patterns are considered to be biological rhythms, since

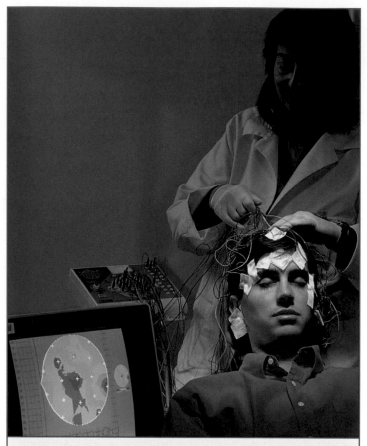

Figure 1.2 The stages of sleep are measured by a device called an **electroencephalograph**, or EEG. When small electrodes are pasted to the scalp and attached to an amplifier, they pick up tiny changes in the electrical activity of the brain. These "brain waves" are plotted on polygraph paper (as used during a lie detector test) or fed directly into a computer and can be analyzed according to their individual characteristics. Brain waves during waking are very small and close together, but in Stage 4 of non-REM sleep the waves become very big and further apart. For this reason, non-REM sleep is often called *slow wave sleep*, because the brain waves on an EEG appear to be slower in their frequency. However, the patterns of brain waves in waking and in REM sleep are strikingly similar.

they repeat each day at approximately the same time (they are also sometimes called **circadian rhythms**, coming from the Latin words *circa dia* meaning "about a day"). We have many biological rhythms—our hormone levels rise and fall during the day in a regular pattern, our blood pressure changes as a function of time of day, and even our mental abilities show some daily patterns (some people are better thinkers in the morning, others in the evening).

These biological rhythms are thought to be controlled by the brain (actually a cluster of approximately 10,000 nerve cells in the brain called the *suprachiasmatic nuclei*). However, biological rhythms are also strongly controlled by external factors such as light. Indeed, people who live in countries lying toward the poles of the earth (i.e., Norway and Iceland) have very different biological rhythms than those who live closer to the equator. For example, because the earth's axis is slightly tilted, during the summers in Iceland there is almost continuous daylight, and during the winter there is often just five hours of light per day. This increased or decreased exposure to daylight causes biological rhythms to differ greatly from those in people who live with the daylight patterns closer to the equator.

WHAT IS THE PURPOSE OF SLEEP?

Why do we sleep? Is its purpose merely to give the body a rest from activity and store up energy? Maybe, but why, then, do we sleep even if we are ill and are forced to stay in bed all day? Or why do newborn babies, even before they are crawling or walking, sleep so much? Maybe infants need to sleep so much because they are doing so much growing. If so, then why do adults sleep if they are already finished growing? Or, if the function of sleep is to give the body a rest, why is the brain and cardiovascular system so active during REM sleep?

These questions go on and on and have plagued scientists and philosophers alike for decades, if not centuries. The answer is there is no right answer. Sleep may have many functions that differ as a function of age, activity, and health status. Some scientists believe sleep helps us get well when we are fighting illnesses. Others believe sleep plays a role in the structural development of the brain and strengthening the connections between nerve cells. Still others believe sleep helps the brain process and store information it received during the day and may even help make some memories more permanent. But the true function(s) of sleep are still largely unknown.

One thing is for certain, though, sleep is absolutely necessary. The more someone is deprived of sleep, the stronger is the drive to fall asleep. And the sleepier the person gets, the worse his or her moods and mental abilities become. Sleepy people have difficulty concentrating, remembering things, learning new information or tasks, and handling minor irritations, and they have impaired logical reasoning. Think of your body as being like car—you can't run a car 24 hours a day, 7 days a week, without refueling, cooling off, or getting a tune-up and an oil change.

Certain animal species have adapted very interesting features of their sleep. For example, bats, which sleep hanging upside down in a cave, do not experience complete atonia when in REM sleep (otherwise they'd fall). Also, animals such as horses and cows can maintain muscle tone in their legs during REM sleep, since they sleep standing up. But one of the most fascinating facts of animal sleep is that certain species, such as dolphins, whales, and some ducks and birds, have developed unihemispheric sleep. That is, one half (or hemisphere) of their brain can go to sleep while the other half remains awake to allow the animal to function normally. But, because half of the brain is inactive, the animal loses the function of that half and has to swim or paddle in a circle using the active half of the brain. Then, after a certain amount of time, they switch hemispheres so the previously active one can sleep. This amazing ability to sleep half of the brain at a time

SLEEP IN OTHER SPECIES

One thing that makes scientists believe sleep is some sort of instinct is the fact that almost all mammals, birds, reptiles, fish, and even insects sleep (or at least rest on a regular basis). Many scientists interested in sleep have turned to the animal kingdom to answer questions about the function of sleep. For instance, why do some animals sleep more than others? What is it about the physiology or behavior of an animal that sleeps a lot or very little that might tell us something about the function of sleep? This question is far from being answered. The chart below lists animals and their average sleep times. Do you know which animal sleeps the most or the least? You may be surprised . . .

Species	Average Sleep Time (total hours per day)
Brown bat	20.0
Opossum	18.0
Python	18.0
Human (infant)	16.0
Tiger	16.0
Three-toed sloth	14.0
Cat	12.0
Mouse	12.0
Bottle-nosed dolphin	10.0
Human (adult)	8.0
Guppy	7.0
Cow	4.0
Elephant	3.5
Horse	3.0
Giraffe	2.0[1]

As you can see, the amount of sleep a particular species needs is not directly proportional to obvious things like its size, number of legs, or whether or not it is nocturnal or diurnal. So, why does a bat need 20 hours of sleep while a giraffe only 2? Your guess is as good as any.

offers these species a tremendous survival advantage and gives new meaning to the phrase "sleep with one eye open."

SLEEP NEEDS CHANGE THROUGHOUT THE LIFE SPAN

It is often said that you need 7–8 hours of sleep: any less and you're not getting enough, any more and you're being lazy. This is one of the most common misconceptions about sleep—that the amount you need is constant across all people. Nothing could further from the truth. The average number of hours of sleep an adult human needs is 7–8 hours per night. And that's all this number is, an average. Some need more, some need less. Some people need only 5–6 hours a night, while others need 9–10 hours. In fact, the amount of sleep a person needs is as individualized as a person's fingerprint. The 19th century inventor Thomas Edison is said to have slept only two hours a night and was once quote as saying that anyone who sleeps more than four hours a night is lazy and a timewaster.

One thing that is true is that the amount of sleep you need changes with age (see Figure 1.3). Babies typically sleep approximately 16 hours per day (often broken up by wet diapers and midnight feedings) and this slowly diminishes to about 8 to 10 hours per day by the time you are a teenager. Unfortunately, most teenagers do not get this amount of sleep because of the demands of school, sports, after school activities, and socializing. In addition, the biological changes that come with adolescence also reset the teenager's biological clock so that he or she is more prone to stay up late and sleep in later. However, most high schools start at 8:00 A.M. or earlier and fail to take into account an adolescent's sleep patterns. As a result, teenagers are often chronically sleep-deprived, falling asleep in class and catching up on lost sleep on the weekends. This chronic sleep deprivation can hinder a teenager's thinking abilities during the day, or when mixed with alcohol, can have very serious consequences.

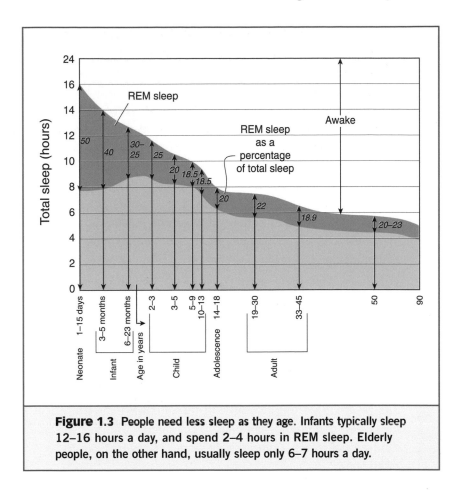

Figure 1.3 People need less sleep as they age. Infants typically sleep 12–16 hours a day, and spend 2–4 hours in REM sleep. Elderly people, on the other hand, usually sleep only 6–7 hours a day.

As mentioned earlier, the average number of hours of sleep needed by an adult is approximately 7 to 8 hours a night. With increasing age, particularly past age 50 or so, the ability to sleep begins to deteriorate and many older people start to experience **insomnia** and frequent nighttime awakenings. In other words, their sleep becomes "fragmented." This often results in sleepiness during the day and the urge to nap. You don't actually need less sleep when you are older, you just aren't able to get the good night's sleep you should.

The amount of time you spend in REM and non-REM sleep also changes with age (refer again to Figure 1.3). Infants

Mike always tended to need a little more sleep than other people his age. Even when he was a baby, he would sleep until 9:00 or 10:00 in the morning, which is quite unusual for an infant. From elementary school through college, Mike always tried to reserve weekend mornings to catch up on lost sleep, often sleeping until 11:00 A.M. or noon. However, once Mike started drinking beer with his buddies in college, he was usually one of the first to pass out after drinking too much. Was he just a lightweight drinker? Actually, no. Alcohol can intensify the effects of sleepiness. So, if you are consistently not getting enough sleep, alcohol can make you sleepier and more prone to fall asleep than if you are getting a full night's rest on a regular basis. Aside from the embarrassment of passing out at parties, this combination of sleep deprivation and alcohol can prove deadly. Both alcohol and sleepiness, alone or in combination, cause thousands of deadly car accidents in high schools and colleges across the United States. In fact, driving while sleepy can be just as dangerous as driving drunk. Studies in humans have shown that sleep deprivation can cause your mental abilities to deteriorate to the same degree as after several drinks of alcohol.

spend 50% or more of their sleep time in REM sleep, which leads scientists to believe that REM sleep plays an important role in the development of the brain and connections between nerve cells. By the time you are 3–5 years old, only about 20% of your sleep time is spent in REM, and this percentage holds steady up through age 50 or so. However, as mentioned before, sleep in the elderly becomes fragmented and the amount of time spent in REM decreases further to about 10%–15% of total sleep.[2]

PERILS OF SLEEP DEPRIVATION

Over the past few decades, sleep deprivation has become a nationwide problem in the United States. With our schedules full of things like homework, sports, jobs, school club meetings and activities, socializing with friends, dating, and family commitments, we often sacrifice an hour or two (or more) of sleep to squeeze in a few extra activities. With cable TV and movie channels available 24 hours a day, supermarkets open around the clock, and the Internet available whenever you want, we have become a society in which, unfortunately, sleep takes a back seat to our other wants and needs.

Although society tolerates this "sleep is for sissies" attitude, scientists and medical professionals are trying hard to educate the public that chronic sleep loss is a serious health issue. It may seem like just some heavy eyelids during class here and a yawn there, but sleep deprivation is indeed very dangerous. Not only does it cause us to be irritable and less tolerant (and perhaps less pleasant to be around), but it also hampers our creative and analytical thinking, physical performance (we run and swim better and lift more weight when we are well-rested), and often leads to health problems like increased susceptibility to colds and infections. If you are still in doubt as to the importance of getting enough sleep, consider these facts:

- The National Highway Traffic Safety Administration estimates that over 200,000 automobile crashes are caused by drowsy drivers every year, resulting in over 1,500 deaths, 70,000 injuries, and an estimated $12.5 billion in lost productivity and property loss. The National Sleep Foundation's 2002 Sleep in America poll showed that over half of Americans said they have driven while feeling drowsy, and approximately 17% said they had actually fallen asleep while driving.[3]

- Driver fatigue causes 30%–40% of all large truck accidents.

- In a recent North Carolina study focusing on car crashes that were caused by the driver falling asleep at the wheel, 55% of the drivers were less than age 25, 78% of the drivers were males, and the most common age of the driver was 20.

- Sleep deprivation was determined to play a role in the 1989 Exxon Valdez oil tanker disaster, the 1986 decision to launch the Space Shuttle Challenger which exploded shortly after takeoff, and numerous deadly commercial airline crashes.

- Doctors are often forced to work 36-hour shifts during their medical residency, and going this long without a good night's rest has resulted in countless medical errors during surgeries or other life-threatening procedures.

- The devastating accidents at the Chernobyl and Three Mile Island nuclear power plants both occurred as a result of erroneous decisions made between the hours of midnight and 3:00 A.M.

SLEEP, THE BRAIN, AND NEUROTRANSMITTERS

Sleep is primarily controlled by the brain (Figure 1.4). Experiments in animals and humans have shown that the brain stem, primarily regions called the **pons** and **medulla**, are largely involved in generating sleep and orchestrating the cycling between the various stages of non-REM sleep, REM sleep, and waking. Also within these regions of the brain stem are centers that control basic bodily functions like heart rate, blood pressure, and breathing, supporting the notion that sleep is a basic instinct and a core bodily function like breathing. These sleep-regulating centers in the brain stem

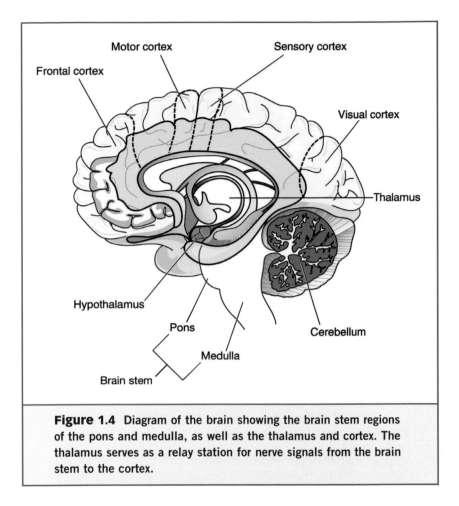

Figure 1.4 Diagram of the brain showing the brain stem regions of the pons and medulla, as well as the thalamus and cortex. The thalamus serves as a relay station for nerve signals from the brain stem to the cortex.

send activating or deactivating signals to the cerebral cortex (the area of the brain where thinking, cognition, and consciousness are believed to occur) via a relay station called the **thalamus**, which also relays all incoming information from most of the five senses. Thus, the brain stem can switch these cycles off and on throughout the various stages of sleeping and waking. The **hypothalamus** is another region that controls sleep and biological rhythms.

Under normal circumstances, **neurons** (nerve cells in the brain) carry electrical signals along wire-like nerve fibers called axons. At the end of each axon is a mushroom-shaped nerve ending called a synaptic terminal. When the electrical signal from the axon reaches the synaptic terminal, it causes chemical messengers called **neurotransmitters** to be released and secreted onto nearby neurons. This junction between a synaptic terminal and a nearby neuron is called a synapse (there are literally millions of synapses in the brain, and each neuron can have as many as 10,000 different synapses on it). After neurotransmitters are released, they diffuse away from the synaptic terminal into the synapse and encounter proteins (called receptors) on the nearby neurons that are designed to recognize specific neurotransmitters. These receptors can cause the nearby nerve cell to either become activated (i.e., it passes along the electrical signal) or inhibited (i.e., it doesn't pass the signal along).

There are dozens of types of neurotransmitters that nerve cells can secrete. One of the main neurotransmitters in the brain is called serotonin. Other common neurotransmitters include dopamine, glutamate, gamma aminobutyric acid (GABA), noradrenaline, and histamine.

Drugs that alter sleep produce their effects on the brain by altering the actions of neurotransmitters and consequently how neurons communicate with each other. However, different drugs can alter the actions of neurotransmitters in different ways. Stimulants such as amphetamine cause neurons to release excess amounts of neurotransmitters like dopamine and serotonin. Other drugs, such as the prescription sleeping pills Halcion® or Ambien® or antihistamines, can interact directly with the neurons' receptors to either enhance or block the effects of the neurotransmitters. In later chapters, we will discuss how drugs that help you sleep or stay awake alter the chemistry of the brain.

2

Sleep Disorders

The brain and its infinite complexity will surely puzzle us for centuries to come. But, as with any other organ in the body, things can go wrong with the brain (and the behavior it controls). Whether it is Alzheimer's or Parkinson's disease, anxiety, depression, or schizophrenia, there is no shortage of possible diseases and disorders of the brain. And sleep, which the brain closely controls and monitors, is also susceptible to going out of whack. In recent decades, with the advancement of sleep research and improved knowledge about sleep, scientists and medical doctors have come to realize that sleep disorders are much more common than anyone previously imagined. In this chapter, we discuss some of the more common sleep disorders, such as insomnia and sleep apnea, as well as more rare disorders like narcolepsy and REM behavior disorder.

INSOMNIA

"The worst thing in the world is to try to sleep and not to."
—**F. Scott Fitzgerald, author of** *The Great Gatsby*

Contrary to popular opinion, insomnia is not just the inability to fall asleep. Insomnia is actually defined as difficulty falling asleep or getting back to sleep after waking in the middle of the night (Figure 2.1). Insomnia always results in poor sleep and usually sleepiness during the following day. Insomnia is usually acute, for only a night or two or just a few weeks, but in some people it can be chronic, lasting three months or longer.

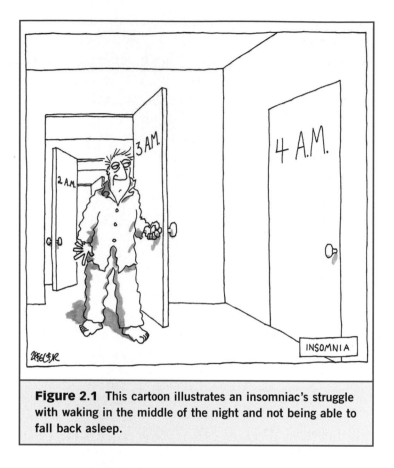

Figure 2.1 This cartoon illustrates an insomniac's struggle with waking in the middle of the night and not being able to fall back asleep.

Insomnia is, by far, the most common sleep disorder: it is estimated that approximately half of adults experience some form of insomnia at least once in their lives. Insomnia is less common in children and teenagers than in adults, but it is particularly prevalent in elderly people, as their sleep becomes "fragmented" with age. Insomnia is slightly more common in females than males.

What causes insomnia? Many things, it turns out, which is perhaps why it is so common. The number one cause of insomnia is stress, whether over an exam, school activity, personal relationship, or family and work issues. Insomnia can also be caused by anxiety or depression, illnesses such as arthritis or other forms of chronic pain, travel across time zones (jet lag), and poor sleep habits (such as drinking caffeine or alcohol, or exercising too close to bedtime). Finally, some medications, such as those used to treat Attention Deficit/Hyperactivity Disorder (ADHD), high blood pressure, or nasal congestion, also interfere with the ability to fall asleep.

Insomnia can have a serious impact on a person's quality of life. Acute insomnia can lead to daytime sleepiness and reduced ability to concentrate, remember things, use logical reasoning, and even impair your ability to drive a car. Chronic insomnia can have major health consequences, such as an increased susceptibility to depression and some forms of heart disease and a reduced ability to fight off colds or infections. There is also a tremendous cost to society caused by insomnia—billions of dollars are spent each year on treatment, healthcare services, and hospital costs. An equal cost can be attributed to lost productivity at work and property and personal damage from accidents caused by sleepy insomniacs.

So how is insomnia treated? Most commonly, people self-medicate their insomnia with over-the-counter medications such as Tylenol PM®, Sominex®, Unisom®, or other drugs such as antihistamines (discussed in Chapter 3). Other people try natural remedies such as melatonin (see Chapter 4). When such medications don't work, people often ask their doctor for a prescription sleep aid, which is usually a type of medication called a benzodiazepine such as Halcion or a related type of drug such as Ambien or Sonata® (see Chapter 6 for more on these types of drugs).

Insomnia can also be treated without medication. This type of treatment is called a behavioral treatment or modification since it is meant to modify the behavior of the insomnia sufferer. One commonly used behavioral treatment is called stimulus control: the person stops doing non-sleep-related activities in bed, such as writing a letter, talking on the phone, studying, or playing computer games. When these types of activities are performed in bed, your brain associates bedtime with these stimulating activities. When they are done at a desk or elsewhere and your bed is used primarily for sleep, your brain associates sleep with bedtime, and thus it becomes easier to fall asleep. Similarly, the insomnia sufferer should get out of bed whenever he or she is not sleeping. This includes not lying awake in bed at night or in the morning for more than 15 minutes. These behavior modifications strengthen the association your brain makes between sleeping and being in bed.

SLEEP APNEA

Once thought to be a rare sleep disorder, **sleep apnea** is actually fairly common, although it often goes undiagnosed by doctors. Sleep apnea was first described as a medical condition in the 1960s, and the term *apnea* is the Greek word meaning "want of breath." Sleep apnea is actually a breathing disorder characterized by brief interruptions of breathing during sleep. There are two types of sleep apnea: central sleep apnea, which is less common and caused by the brain's failure to send proper signals to the muscles involved in breathing, and obstructive sleep apnea, which is much more common and is caused by the tongue or excess tissue in the back of the throat blocking the airways (see Figure 2.2).

People with sleep apnea typically have 20 to 60 apneic events (interruptions in breathing) per hour of sleep. The interruptions in breathing cause levels of oxygen in the blood to drop and levels of carbon dioxide to rise. These changes in the blood send a signal to the brain that causes the person to arouse from sleep and start breathing again, but usually the person does not wake up all the way to full consciousness. The brain also sends a signal to the airway muscles to open and restore normal breathing, usually resulting in some kind of a gasp or snort.

Because of these apneic events, a sleep apnea sufferer never really enters the deep, restorative stages of sleep. In fact, the person is aroused from sleep numerous times per hour and,

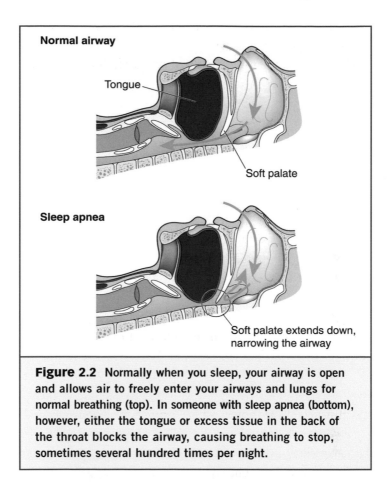

Normal airway

Tongue

Soft palate

Sleep apnea

Soft palate extends down,
narrowing the airway

Figure 2.2 Normally when you sleep, your airway is open
and allows air to freely enter your airways and lungs for
normal breathing (top). In someone with sleep apnea (bottom),
however, either the tongue or excess tissue in the back of
the throat blocks the airway, causing breathing to stop,
sometimes several hundred times per night.

hence, is never able to get a good night's rest. The result is often
that the person is extremely sleepy during the day. In addition to
daytime sleepiness, there are also more severe health consequences
of sleep apnea: the constant interruptions in breathing often result
in cardiovascular problems, such as irregular heartbeat, high
blood pressure, and an increased risk of heart attack or stroke.

It is estimated that approximately 18 million people in the
United States suffer from sleep apnea. The disorder occurs
slightly more often in males than in females and is also more
common in overweight people, probably because these people
tend to have more build up of fatty tissue in the throat, which

increases the likelihood of the airway becoming blocked during sleep. In addition, if a person with sleep apnea drinks alcohol or takes a sleeping pill prior to bedtime, this can increase the duration of each apneic event and make the cardiovascular consequences of the disorder much worse.

As a result of these constant awakenings and the failure to get needed deep, restorative sleep, the sleep apnea sufferer is often very fatigued during the day, has difficulty with learning and memory, and may become depressed and irritable. Because these people are so tired during the day, they often fall asleep at work or at school and are three times more likely to have an automobile accident.

Sleep apnea is not usually treated with medications, although medications may be prescribed to treat the associated high blood pressure or irregular heartbeat associated with the disorder. The following is a list of possible treatments for sleep apnea:

- Use of a breathing apparatus known as a **CPAP (continuous positive airway pressure**) device. This is the most common and effective method for treating sleep apnea. The patient wears a mask over the nose during sleep, which constantly and gently pumps air through the nasal passages. The result of the continuous air flow is that the airways remain open and breathing is not interrupted.

- Use of dental appliances that reposition the lower jaw and tongue so it does not block the airways during sleep.

- Surgical removal of the excess tissue at the back of the throat.

- In more severe and life-threatening instances of sleep apnea, a tracheostomy is performed, in which a hole is drilled into the windpipe through the front of the neck and a tube is inserted to allow air to enter and exit the

SNORING—IS IT NORMAL OR A SIGN OF A SLEEP DISORDER?

"Laugh and the world laughs with you; snore and you sleep alone."

—Anthony Burgess,
author of *Clockwork Orange*

We all snore or know someone who does. We often laugh and make jokes about people who snore. In cartoons, the sound of snoring is often depicted by a string of ZZZs. And sleeping in the same room with someone who snores can be quite a challenge.

We snore because when we inhale air during sleep, the tissue at the back of the throat (called the soft palate) and the uvula (that odd dangling thing at the back of your mouth) can vibrate and produce noise. The volume of someone's snoring varies greatly, depending on the amount and speed of the air passing through and the person's sleeping position (sleeping on your back causes the tongue and tissue to fall against the very back of your throat, increasing the likelihood of snoring).

In some people, snoring is completely harmless and doesn't impair breathing. But in others, snoring may be a sign of a serious health problem. Snoring is often a sign of sleep apnea, since the tissue causing the snoring can be blocking the airway and causing an interruption of breathing. Like sleep apnea, snoring is often more common in overweight people and those who drink alcohol before bedtime (because alcohol tends to relax muscles and tissue in the throat). In addition, people who breathe primarily through their mouth (either by habit or because of allergies and nasal congestion) also tend to snore. Weight loss, avoiding alcohol, and sleeping on one's side can help reduce the incidence of snoring.

lungs. During waking hours, the tube is plugged and the person breathes normally, but during sleep the person breathes through the tube rather than his or her mouth and nose.

- Behavioral modifications such as weight loss, avoidance of alcohol and sleeping pills, and the use of specialized pillows that encourage the person to sleep on his or her side (sleep apnea occurs most often when the person is sleeping on his or her back).

NARCOLEPSY

Despite its name, the sleep disorder **narcolepsy** does not have anything to do with narcotics or epilepsy. Narcolepsy is a bizarre and relatively rare sleep disorder, affecting approximately one out of every 2,000 people. Originally, doctors described narcoleptic patients as suffering from sudden and uncontrollable "sleep attacks," where a person falls asleep while eating at the dinner table or in the middle of making a speech. Doctors attributed narcolepsy to not getting enough sleep at night, and some even thought it was some form of seizure.

However, it turns out that narcolepsy is a complex sleep disorder that is primarily genetic in nature (i.e., it runs in families). Narcolepsy affects both males and females alike. There are several main symptoms of narcolepsy. Usually the first to appear is extreme sleepiness during the daytime, no matter how much sleep the person gets at night. The person repeatedly feels an intense urge to fall asleep at many times throughout the day. Without proper medication, people with narcolepsy often find it almost impossible to stay awake for more than an hour or two. These urges to sleep are often accompanied by a symptom called **cataplexy**, where the person suddenly loses muscle tone in his or her arms, legs, face, or neck. The person's arms and legs may just get temporarily weak, or the person can actually collapse entirely. This is the same muscle "paralysis" that you experience normally at night when you enter REM sleep (as discussed in Chapter 1). When a person has an attack of cataplexy, he or she can remain awake (but partially or fully unable to move) or immediately enter REM sleep and start dreaming (recall from Chapter 1 that when we go to sleep at night, we normally experience 60–90 minutes of non-REM sleep before we enter REM sleep). In other words, people with narcolepsy actually experience "attacks" of REM sleep. They may be talking or reading one moment, and the next they may fall directly into REM sleep, which as we know is where dreaming takes place and the skeletal muscles are temporarily paralyzed.

Oddly, the most common triggers for cataplexy are laughter, anger, fear, surprise, or other strong emotions. So, while most of us bend over with laughter after hearing a really funny joke, patients with narcolepsy can actually collapse to the ground and directly enter REM sleep. And, since brief episodes of REM sleep often occur during these attacks of cataplexy, the patient can be awake one moment and dreaming the next. Imagine that while you are reading this book in a chair, you suddenly hear a door slam, which startles you and causes you to fall directly into REM sleep and you dream that the words on the page start to move around or speak to you. Then you suddenly recover from the attack of cataplexy and awaken to find yourself having dropped the book and fallen out of the chair. This rapid sequence of entering and exiting REM sleep causes the narcoleptic patient to experience what are called **hypnagogic hallucinations**, which are bizarre and often frightening dreams and sounds that occur during the onset or waking up from cataplexy. Sometimes people with narcolepsy who experience these hallucinations have difficulty determining what is real and what is dreamed.

Similar to cataplexy, people with narcolepsy often experience sleep paralysis, which is the inability to move or talk for a brief period upon going to sleep or waking up. This sleep paralysis is the same that you experience while in REM sleep. However, in people with narcolepsy, sleep paralysis often occurs in conjunction with hypnagogic hallucinations. So, the patient may be awoken from sleep and be unable to move, while at the same time experiencing a terrifying hallucination that a person with a knife is chasing him, and he are unable to try and run or defend himself (even though it is just a dream-like image).

Because most of the symptoms of narcolepsy are characteristics of REM sleep, the disorder is often viewed as "intrusions" of REM sleep into wakefulness. Scientists believe that the regions in the brain that control REM sleep are malfunctioning in the patient with narcolepsy, sending erroneous signals to other parts of the brain and the rest of the body to enter REM sleep when it is not appropriate. This makes the narcoleptic individual have difficulty separating wakefulness from REM sleep and non-REM sleep. In addition, the fact that emotions are the primary trigger of cataplexy makes scientists believe that brain regions involved in controlling emotions (these brain regions are collectively known as the **limbic system**) may have faulty connections with the brain regions that control REM sleep.

The first symptoms of narcolepsy usually appear between the ages of 15 and 30. Unfortunately, narcolepsy is a lifelong disorder for which there are not yet effective cures. Narcolepsy is primarily treated with medications to control the symptoms (many of these are discussed in Chapter 5). Strong prescription stimulants such as dextroamphetamine (Dexedrine®), methylphenidate (Ritalin®), and pemoline (Cylert®) are often used to combat the excessive sleepiness in narcoleptic patients. A non-stimulant medication called modafinil (Provigil®) was recently approved by the U.S. Food and Drug Administration for controlling sleepiness in narcolepsy. Other symptoms of narcolepsy, such as cataplexy, hypnagogic hallucinations, and sleep paralysis, are controlled with antidepressants such as imipramine (Tofranil®), desimpramine (Norpramin®), chlomipramine (Anafranil®), protriptyline (Vivactil®), fluoxetine (Prozac®), paroxetine (Paxil®), and sertraline (Zoloft®). Since the nighttime sleep of narcoleptic patients is fragmented (likely because the brain mechanisms controlling sleep are not functioning properly), these patients are sometimes prescribed a newer medication called sodium oxybate (Xyrem®). Xyrem is very sedating and is only taken at night to help the patient get a better, more restful night's sleep.

Because narcoleptics are prone to fall sleep or lose muscle control very quickly, they often have difficulty in school and work and are certainly recommended to limit their time spent driving (some states even prohibit narcoleptics from driving altogether). So, significant lifestyle changes must be adapted by the narcoleptic patient, such as joining support groups, finding rides to and from school or social events, avoiding cataplexy triggers (such as funny movies), trying to schedule regular naps, scheduling classes around the times of day when the patient is most sleepy, and finding friends to borrow class notes from or audiotaping lectures. Narcoleptic individuals are often depressed about their condition and may become socially withdrawn and experience loss of self-esteem. In addition, medication side effects may cause a loss of interest in sex or reduced sexual performance.

RESTLESS LEGS SYNDROME

Restless legs syndrome, or RLS, is a sleep disorder in which a person feels an irresistible urge to move his or her legs to alleviate creeping, crawling, tingling, cramping, or painful feelings in the legs. This is not just the occasional tightness or cramping you might feel if you are a runner, soccer player, or other athlete that uses his or her legs a lot. These urges are always worse at night or when the person is lying down. The urge to move the legs is irresistible and constant throughout

(continued on page 36)

NARCOLEPTIC DOGS HELP SCIENTISTS DISCOVER THE CAUSE OF NARCOLEPSY

Since animals sleep, this begs the question—do animals have sleep disorders? Well, we may never know if animals suffer from insomnia because we can't ask them, "Are you getting enough sleep?" But in fact, there are several species of animals that display behaviors remarkably similar to symptoms of human sleep disorders. For example, pigs can show signs of sleep apnea and have been used to study potential treatments for the disorder.

One of the most striking findings of an apparent sleep disorder in animals is the narcoleptic dogs studied at Stanford University. In the 1970s, sleep research pioneers Dr. William Dement and Dr. Christian Guilleminault, who started the world's first sleep disorders clinic at Stanford, came across several breeds of dogs, including poodles and Doberman pinschers that appeared to have narcolepsy. The dogs would at times appear very drowsy while standing, and if given food (which normally gets dogs very excited), they would lose control over their neck and leg muscles and often collapse. Dr. Dement and Dr. Guilleminault started breeding these dogs to maintain a colony of them for research. They eventually connected these dogs to an EEG and found that they suffered attacks of cataplexy and immediately entered REM sleep if they got too excited when given food.

The narcoleptic dogs at Stanford were further studied at both Stanford and the University of California at Los Angeles throughout the 1970s, 1980s, and 1990s. Scientists tested potential medications for treatment and performed genetic analysis of these dogs with the hope of finding a genetic cause of the disorder. Then, in the late 1990s, a brilliant researcher at Stanford named Dr. Emmanuel Mignot (Figure 2.3) made a landmark breakthrough when he discovered that narcoleptic dogs carried a mutated gene that disrupted the production of a neurotransmitter called hypocretin, which we

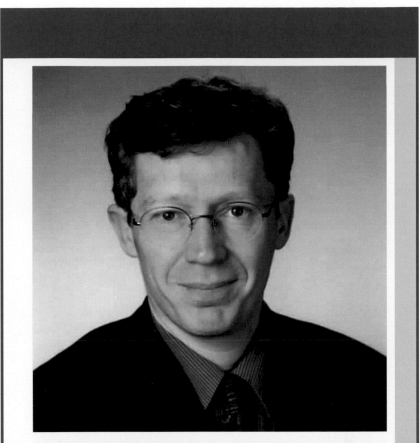

Figure 2.3 *Dr. Emmanuel Mignot of Stanford University discov-ered that narcoleptic dogs carried a mutated gene which disrupted the production of hypocretin.*

now know is an active controller of wakefulness and the various stages of REM sleep. Subsequent studies in mice bred with this mutated gene showed that these mice had signs of narcolepsy, confirming that the lack of hypocretin is the primary problem in narcolepsy. As a result of these important animal studies, medications based on replacing this neurotransmitter are now being developed to treat narcolepsy, and scientists are hoping to develop genetic tests to determine who might be susceptible to developing narcolepsy.

(continued from page 33)
the night and, as a result, it severely disrupts the person's sleep. Moving, bending, stretching, rubbing the legs, or getting up and pacing back and forth are the only way to relieve these urges, and the relief is only temporary.

It is estimated that RLS affects up to 10% of the population in North America and Europe. In Japan, India, and Singapore, the rates of incidence are much lower, suggesting that ethnic factors may play a role in the disorder. RLS also tends to run in families, suggesting a genetic basis. RLS affects males and females alike, and the symptoms seem to get worse as the person grows older. Pregnancy and hormonal changes also make the symptoms of RLS worse. The severity of the symptoms can rise and fall over time and may even occasionally temporarily disappear.

The cause of RLS is still unknown, but likely involves a deficiency in the neurotransmitter dopamine. Scientists suspect a dopamine deficiency is to blame because the most widely prescribed medication for treating RLS is levadopa (also called L-dopa), which the body turns into dopamine. Other medications that seem to alleviate symptoms are opiate drugs such as codeine and oxycodone, but these must only be administered occasionally since they are prone to cause addiction. Finally, some benzodiazepines (discussed in Chapter 6) also help the RLS sufferer get a better night's rest.

PERIODIC LIMB MOVEMENTS IN SLEEP
Similar to RLS, **periodic limb movements in sleep** (**PLMS**) is a sleep disorder in which people move their limbs (particularly the legs) during sleep. In PLMS, a person involuntarily twitches their legs every 20 to 40 seconds while sleeping. The difference between PLMS and RLS is that PLMS patients do not always feel the crawling uncomfortable sensations that make them want to move their legs. The limb movements in PLMS often occur during sleep while the person is completely unaware of them. However, occasionally PLMS can cause the person to

wake up during the movements, resulting in poor sleep and subsequently daytime sleepiness.

PLMS occurs mostly in older people, with an estimated 35% or more of elderly people suffering from the disorder. It can also occur in younger people and seems to affect males and females equally. Occasionally, PLMS has been associated with other medical problems such as kidney disease or diabetes. The cause of PLMS is unknown, but like RLS it may involve a dopamine deficiency. PLMS is usually treated with the same types of medications as for RLS (see above).

NIGHTMARES AND SLEEP TERRORS

You have probably had a nightmare at least once in your lifetime. **Nightmares** are vivid dreams with very disturbing content that often cause the person to wake up. They occur more frequently in children and usually during REM sleep, when most dreams occur. Nightmares are almost always remembered.

Sleep terrors, sometimes called night terrors, are often mistakenly described as nightmares, and they also occur mostly in children. During a sleep terror, the person appears to wake up screaming and terrified and may cry inconsolably for several minutes. However, often the person is not fully awake during the night terror. The sufferer often shows several physical signs of fear, such as sweating, dilated pupils, and increased blood pressure. After several minutes of a night terror, the person then calms down and returns to sleep. Unlike nightmares, however, sleep terrors occur primarily during non-REM sleep (when dreaming does not normally occur), so it is not likely that the terror is in response to a bad dream. In addition, unlike nightmares, a person rarely recalls what he or she experienced or sometimes only has a vague memory of some frightening images.

Sleep terrors are a type of sleep disorder known as a parasomnia (abnormal physical behavior during sleep) that occur mostly in children but can happen at any age. They are typically just a few minutes long but can last up to 10–20 minutes. They tend to run in families and are usually treated with benzodiazepines such as Klonopin® and Valium® (see Chapter 6) or the antidepressant imipramine (Tofranil).

SLEEPWALKING AND SLEEPTALKING

Sleepwalking (also called somnambulism) and **sleeptalking** (also called somniloquy) are parasomnias that primarily affect children but occur in adults as well (affecting as much as 15% of the population). Contrary to popular belief, people who sleepwalk are not acting out their dreams (remember your muscles are paralyzed during REM sleep; people who act out their dreams have REM behavior disorder, discussed later in this chapter). Sleepwalking is when a person typically sits up and gets out of bed with a "glazed" look in his eyes and moves around the room with clumsy or purposeless movements. Sleepwalkers may even engage in complex behaviors such as getting dressed or undressed, going to the bathroom, drawing objects on the wall, going out of the room or even the house, and have even been reported to get in their cars and drive as far as getting on the freeway. Sleepwalking episodes can last from 15 seconds to 30 minutes and usually occur during the first episode of Stage 4 non-REM sleep of the night. Sleepwalkers generally do not respond to voices but can be led by the hand back to bed. Sleepwalkers rarely recall the event, and unless they routinely engage in some sort of behavior that is dangerous (i.e., operating a car, climbing onto the roof, etc.), there is no need for medical treatment. Problem sleepwalkers are usually treated with a benzodiazepine such as Klonopin.

Sleeptalking can occur at any age and is more common in females than males. Sleeptalking is characterized by either nonsense babbling or mumbling a few words, and at times the person can utter complete coherent sentences. Sleeptalking usually occurs in Stages 1 or 2 of non-REM sleep but has occasionally been known to occur in REM sleep where the person utters what he or she is saying in his or her dreams. Sleeptalking is usually of little medical concern and very rarely requires treatment.

SLEEP BRUXISM (TEETH GRINDING)

Sleep bruxism is fairly common and characterized by clenching of the jaw and/or grinding of the teeth during sleep without the person's awareness. It is estimated that 5% to 20% of the population shows some form of sleep bruxism. The teeth grinding is actually quite loud and unpleasant and can wake someone else in the room sleeping 10 to 20 feet away. The teeth grinding episodes occur in regular intervals for 4 to 5 seconds and can occur 25 times or more during the night. Sleep bruxism is not confined to a particular stage of sleep. The sleeper is unaware of the problem and may awaken in the morning with sore jaw muscles. When sleep bruxism is a chronic problem, the tops of the teeth (particularly the molars) can wear down and cause various dental problems. Dentists are usually the first to notice if a person has sleep bruxism. To reduce potential damage to the teeth, dentists usual have the patient wear a mouthguard of some sort at night.

SLEEP-RELATED EATING DISORDER

This disorder is not the occasional waking up hungry and going for a midnight snack. **Sleep-related eating disorder** is actually a kind of sleepwalking where the person gets up (after falling asleep), goes to the kitchen, and proceeds to eat a substantial amount of food, then returns to bed and awakens the next morning with no memory of it. Imagine putting leftover pizza in your fridge at night and the next morning you wake up with cheese and tomato sauce on your face and shirt. Even worse, imagine finding an empty package of raw chicken on the kitchen floor.

People with sleep-related eating disorder, which is considered a parasomnia, often find they have unusual weight gain and can develop a fear of choking or starting a fire (on the stove) while eating during sleep. They also feel as if they have lost control over their sleep and eating habits. After they come to realize they may have a problem, people with this disorder often try various methods to stop themselves from eating after going to sleep, such as putting a lock or warning signs on the refrigerator or pantry door or even locking themselves in their bedroom.

Sleep-related eating disorder begins in one's teens or early twenties, and approximately two-thirds of the people who suffer from the disorder are female. Almost 75% of those who have the disorder eat during sleep every night, sometimes up to eight times a night. The vast majority of people who suffer from this disorder are completely unaware of or only partially aware of their own sleep eating habits. Most people with sleep-related eating disorders do not have daytime eating disorders such as anorexia or bulimia.

What causes this bizarre sleep disorder? Well, it doesn't appear to be hunger. Sometimes it can be induced by taking an antidepressant medication, quitting alcohol or smoking, severe stress or childhood trauma, or an infection of the brain. It is typically treated with the same types of medications used to treat RLS or PLMS, such as benzodiazepines, dopamine-replacing drugs, or opiates like oxycodone. In addition, if the underlying cause is some sort of psychological issue, counseling or psychotherapy can also be quite useful.

REM BEHAVIOR DISORDER

Another bizarre parasomnia we mentioned earlier is known as **REM behavior disorder** (**RBD**), sometimes called REM without atonia. In this disorder, when the brain enters REM sleep, it does not send the proper signal to the skeletal muscles to temporarily paralyze you while you dream. The result is that people actually act out portions of their dream or the dream in its entirety! If the person dreams he or she is kicking a soccer ball, he or she may actually kick his or her foot and hit the wall next to the bed, or even his or her bed partner. If the person dreams he is boxing, he may actually throw a punch or two. Other behaviors include talking, shouting, screaming, or even leaping out of bed, all in concert with whatever the person is dreaming about. Obviously, for people who sleep alone, there is a risk of injury from hitting walls or nightstands. For RBD patients who have a bed partner, they usually wake up to the patient's flailing around and either try to defend themselves or wake up the RBD patient. In experiments with cats, when the brain region that regulates muscle atonia during REM sleep was lesioned or destroyed, the cats showed behavior like RBD patients, acting out the dreams by hissing, arching their backs, or chasing a mouse around the room, all while apparently in REM sleep.

Unless they come into contact with something or someone and are awakened, people with REM behavior disorder are unaware that they are acting out their dreams. For those who only act out part of their dream, there is no telling which part will just be kept inside the person's head and which will be acted out. Interestingly, most people who suffer from RBD are generally calm and friendly during the day and do not appear to have violent tendencies.

More than 90% of RBD patients are male and usually older than 50, although sometimes it can be seen in children, teens, and young adults. Fortunately, RBD is relatively rare (occurring in less than 1% of the population) and is effectively treated with the benzodiazepine clonazepam (Klonopin).

Doctors have found an association between taking certain antidepressants, such as Paxil, Zoloft, Prozac, and Celexa®, for depression or anxiety problems and the presence of RBD symptoms. For reasons still unknown, the chemical changes in the brain that antidepressants exert to relieve depression or anxiety can also cause people to have RBD.

When Sean was 19 and a freshman in college, he started to have anxiety problems. He would feel scared a lot of the time for no particular reason. His mind was preoccupied by worrying about little or absurd things, he had difficulty concentrating, and he started to have bad dreams. He realized his anxiety was excessive but thought the problem would just go away on its own. When it didn't go away after a few years, he decided to see a psychiatrist to determine if anything could be done to alleviate the anxiety.

The psychiatrist prescribed Paxil, and although within a few months his anxiety started to subside, he started to have brief periods during sleep when he would act out his dreams. One time, he dreamed that he was fighting off an attacking dog and punched the table lamp next to his bed. Another time, he dreamed he was a kicker for a football team and when he went to kick the opening kickoff, he actually kicked the wall

JET LAG

One last sleep "disorder" that all of us experience (except those who don't travel) is actually a temporary maladaptation of the brain and body's biological rhythms. **Jet lag** occurs when we travel to a new time zone and our biological rhythms are slow to catch up and adjust to the new sunrise and sunset times. As mentioned in Chapter 1, our sleep and biological rhythms are intricately tied to the daily cycles of light and dark.

For example, if your normal bedtime is 10:00 P.M., you and your body are used to going to bed 3–4 hours after the sun next to his bed and stubbed his big toe pretty hard. Sean never recalled experiencing these events before he started taking Paxil.

He would vaguely remember these experiences in the morning, but didn't think too much of them. That was until he got married and started sharing a bed with his wife. Although these events would only happen once every few weeks, there were times he smacked his wife in the face with his hand and elbowed her pretty hard in the ribs. Needless to say, she did not think it was very funny and suggested Sean talk to his doctor about it. Sure enough, the doctor knew that people taking antidepressants like Paxil were likely to develop RBD. Sean's doctor also prescribed Klonopin, and now Sean rarely acts out his dreams.

Of course, Sean could have just stopped taking the Paxil to see if the problem would go away, but fortunately his doctor told him that he could have a relapse of anxiety and experience withdrawal symptoms. Stopping any medication should only be done under a doctor's advice and never done suddenly—the medication should always be tapered off by gradually decreasing the dose over a period of weeks or months.

sets. But if you fly from California to New York (a time difference of three hours) and go to bed at your usual time, your body still thinks it is 7:00 P.M. and you may not be able to fall asleep for another three hours. On the other hand, if you have been in New York for several days and are flying back to California, the situation reverses itself. Now, when you try to go to bed at 10:00 P.M. Pacific time, your body's clock tells you it's 1:00 A.M. and you should be as tired as if you had stayed up an extra three hours. The more time zones you travel across, the worse the jet lag becomes: flying to Asia or

Australia, which are 14–18 hours ahead of the United States, wreaks total havoc on the biological clock. Incidentally, jet lag did not exist until the development of commercial air travel, because other forms of travel are too slow to cause a sudden change in biological rhythms.

So, how do you avoid jet lag? Here are some tips according to the National Sleep Foundation[4]:

- When you arrive at your destination, stay up until at least 10:00 P.M. local time. Don't go to bed too early.

- Don't nap for longer than two hours on the plane, because this throws off your ability to go to sleep later.

- Set an alarm to wake you up at your normal wake-up time locally.

- Anticipate the time change by going to bed a couple of hours earlier for several days prior to flying eastbound or a couple of hours later for a westbound flight.

- When you board the plane, set your watch to the new time at your destination.

- As always, avoid exercise, alcohol, or caffeine (including chocolate) for 3–4 hours prior to bedtime.

- Avoid heavy meals upon arrival at your destination.

- When at your new destination, try to get outside during the day as much as possible—sunlight is an extremely powerful stimulant that resets the biological clock. Staying indoors can worsen jet lag.

3

Over-the-Counter
Sleep Aids

By definition, any medication you can buy at your local pharmacy or grocery store without a prescription—cold medicines, pain relievers, sleep aids—is considered an **over-the-counter** (**OTC**) medication. OTC sleep aids are generally mild enough that most people who use them do not overdose on them or become addicted. However, because anyone can buy OTC sleep aids in any quantity and they are not usually taken under the supervision of a doctor, misuse and abuse of OTC sleep aids can sometimes occur.

ANTIHISTAMINES

The most popular OTC sleep aids are those that contain **antihistamines** such as diphenhydramine or doxylamine (Table 3.1). As noted in Chapter 1, nerve cells in the brain communicate with each other by secreting chemicals called neurotransmitters. One such neurotransmitter that regulates sleep is histamine. When histamine is released by a nerve cell, it diffuses over to the target nerve cell and binds to specialized proteins called receptors located on the outer surface of the nerve cell. These receptors are specially designed to bind only histamine, and when they do, the target nerve cell will become either activated or deactivated. In the brain, histamine serves the function of keeping us awake, and when drugs such as antihistamines are taken, they block the ability of histamine receptors to bind histamine. As a result, histamine is no longer able to maintain its ability to promote wakefulness, and we become drowsy and sleepy.

But histamine also serves a function in the body's immune system. When we have an allergic reaction to something, our immune cells release histamine in the eyes, nose, skin, and airways to cause itchiness, runny nose, sneezing, coughing, and wheezing. It is for this reason we take antihistamines (such as Benadryl®) to control allergy symptoms. However, since histamine has functions in both the brain and the immune system, blocking histamine receptors with antihistamines can relieve allergy symptoms while causing us to become drowsy. This is why pharmaceutical companies have developed newer medications (such as Claritin®, Zyrtec®, Alavert®, and Allegra®) that primarily block histamine action in the immune system and not the brain, preventing the unwanted side effect of drowsiness.

Table 3.1 Common OTC Sleep Aids Containing Antihistamines

BRAND NAME	ACTIVE INGREDIENT
Doan's P.M.*	diphenhydramine
Excedrin P.M.®*	diphenhydramine
Good Night's Sleep® (spray)	diphenhydramine
Nytol®	diphenhydramine
Sleepinal®	diphenhydramine
Sleep-Eze®	diphenhydramine
Sominex®	diphenhydramine
Tylenol P.M.®/Simply Sleep®*	diphenhydramine
Unisom®	doxylamine
Unisom Sleepgels®	diphenhydramine

* These medications are actually pain relievers to which the antihistamine diphenhydramine has been added.

Not everyone reacts to antihistamine-containing sleep aids the same way. Some people, particularly those of Asian descent, are less sensitive to the sedative effects of these medications. Others can have reactions that are opposite to the intended effect of inducing sleepiness—some people feel nervous, jittery, anxious, restless, or agitated after taking antihistamines. This is particularly true in elderly persons and young children. Others can experience a "morning hangover" effect, characterized by sleepiness, headache, dry mouth, constipation, and blurred vision.

HERBAL REMEDIES

Aside from the standard OTC sleep aids, some health food and nutrition stores sell sleep aids that don't contain antihistamines, but rather a cocktail of natural substances such as herbal extracts, amino acids, vitamins, and other ingredients. There are dozens of herbal sleep remedies available, but popular ones include Nite-Rest, Nite-Rite, Sleep-Max®, Sound Sleep®, Deep Sleep®, Great Night Sleep, Mellodyn™, Somnatrol™, Somnulin™, Dromias™, Sleep Aid Herbal Formula, Herbal Sleep, and Herbalist Sleeping Remedy. All of these herbal sleep aids contain a mixture of several of the following herbs, which have been used for centuries to treat a variety of illnesses. (Many of these herbal sleep aids also contain the natural hormone melatonin, which will be discussed in Chapter 4.)

Chamomile (*Matricaria camomilla*): The flowers of this plant are dried and crushed into a tea, and people who drink chamomile tea half an hour or so before bedtime report getting a restful night's sleep. Chamomile tea can be useful for mild insomnia that occurs occasionally. Chamomile contains molecules called flavonoids, particularly chrysin, that calm the activity of nerve cells, although it is unknown exactly how this is achieved. Chamomile can also help relieve anxiety. A note of caution: Since chamomile is a plant like ragweed and chrysanthemum, it produces pollen that, in some people prone to hayfever and other allergies, can cause sneezing.

Kava (*Piper methysticum*): The roots of kava contain molecules called dihydropyrones that help promote muscle relaxation and increased sleep quality. Kava is often incorporated into drinks such as teas or can be taken in capsule form. However, it should be noted that combining kava with alcohol may cause sedation that can cloud thinking and impair the ability to drive a car.

DO'S AND DON'TS OF OTC SLEEP AIDS

It would be tempting to run out and buy a box of OTC sleep aids to have on hand every time it takes you more than 30 minutes to fall asleep or if you are anticipating a stressful time in your life (i.e., final exams) and think you will have trouble sleeping. However, because of the dangers of drug side effects, developing dependence on sleeping pills, and interaction of these medications with other drugs, OTC sleep aids should only be used when absolutely necessary. Here are some do's and don'ts for proper use of OTC sleep aids, particularly those containing antihistamines.

DO:

- Use OTC sleep aids only on occasion, such as for temporary insomnia lasting just a few days or to overcome jet lag.

- See a doctor if your insomnia lasts for more than 7 to 10 days. This may mean you have a more serious sleep problem.

- Read the directions and warnings on the OTC sleep aid package before taking the medication.

- Stick to the recommended dose on the package.

Lavender (*Lavender angustifolia* and other variations): The oil of the lavender plant (Figure 3.1) has been shown to calm the activity of the central nervous system in a fashion similar to stronger prescription tranquilizers, such as benzodiazepines and barbiturates. Lavender is usually put into teas or into candles to create an aroma that is inhaled to produce relaxation and improve the quality of sleep.

Passionflower (*Passiflora incarnate*): Also known as may-pop, passionflower is a woody vine that produces flowers which are picked and dried to produce the passionflower

DON'T:

- Combine OTC sleep aids with alcohol or prescription sleep aids such as benzodiazepines or barbiturates. This can lead to severe sedation, morning sleepiness, hypothermia, and even reduced breathing.

- Take OTC sleep aids containing antihistamines if you are already taking an antihistamine for allergy or cold symptoms. This can increase your risk of antihistamine overdose.

- Take OTC sleep aids if you are pregnant or have a heart condition, constipation, or an enlarged prostate gland.

- Take an OTC sleep aid for more than 7 to 10 nights in a row, as this can result in dependence and addiction.

- Take more than the recommended dose.

- Drive after taking an OTC sleep aid.

- Continue to take the medication if you've experienced a serious side effect.

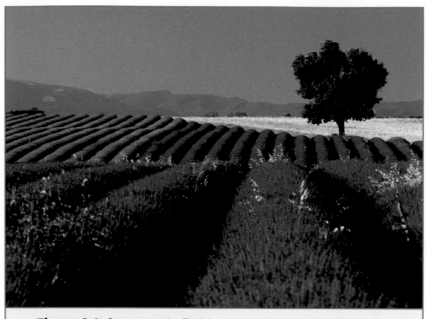

Figure 3.1 Some people find herbal sleep remedies (such as lavender, seen here) to be safe, nontoxic, and healthier alternatives to OTC sleep medications.

extract. Passionflower produces calmness and relaxation while also reducing anxiety, although scientists are not sure precisely how it lowers the activity of the central nervous system.

Valerian (*Valeriana officinalis*): The roots of this plant are dried to produce a potent extract that induces sleepiness and helps treat insomnia. Like lavender, it depresses the activity of the central nervous system in a fashion similar to stronger prescription tranquilizers such as benzodiazepines and barbiturates, but without the dulling or hangover effects the next day or impairing the ability to drive a car.

Some people find herbal sleep remedies to be safe, nontoxic, and healthier alternatives to OTC sleep medications or prescription tranquilizers, such as benzodiazepines and barbiturates. Although generally herbal sleep aids are less potent than prescription medications, they also tend to have fewer side effects, such as dulled thinking and morning hangover, and are much less likely to cause addiction.

However, as with most herbal substances and supplements, the concentration and precise ingredients of herbal sleep remedies are not regulated by the U.S. Food and Drug Administration. Therefore, it is always possible that any one of the herbal products might contain an ingredient that a person is allergic to or otherwise cannot tolerate. Thus, people who use these products should exercise care in the type and amount of these sleep aids that they consume.

4

Melatonin

In recent years, there has been a lot of hype in the media about melatonin and its use as an aid to treat temporary insomnia or jet lag. There has also been some controversy and debate among scientists and physicians as to whether or not melatonin actually helps people sleep. Regardless, melatonin is sold as an over-the-counter supplement in most pharmacies and nutrition and health food stores (Figure 4.1). However, since it is sold as a dietary supplement, the amount of melatonin in each pill as well as the makeup of other ingredients that these melatonin pills might contain, are not regulated by the U.S. Food and Drug Administration.

WHAT IS MELATONIN?

Melatonin is a hormone produced by a gland in the brain called the pineal gland (see Figure 4.2). This gland rests in the center of the brain just above the brainstem. The pineal gland receives information from other regions of the brain involved in biological rhythms, including the master clock of the brain known as the suprachiasmatic nucleus (discussed in Chapter 1), located in the hypothalamus. The pineal gland secretes melatonin into the bloodstream where it can diffuse to other areas of the body and back to the brain. Despite the fact that the brain produces melatonin, many people take melatonin pills to boost levels of the hormone circulating in the blood.

Melatonin is synthesized from the amino acid tryptophan by several enzymes located inside cells in the pineal gland. As seen in Figure 4.3, tryptophan is first converted to 5-hydroxytryptophan

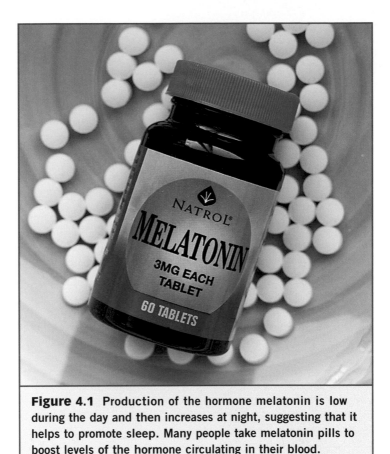

Figure 4.1 Production of the hormone melatonin is low during the day and then increases at night, suggesting that it helps to promote sleep. Many people take melatonin pills to boost levels of the hormone circulating in their blood.

(5-HTP) and then to serotonin (which is also called 5-hydroxy-tryptamine, or 5-HT). **Serotonin** is a neurotransmitter (chemical messenger) that is present in many regions of the brain and is thought to be involved in regulating sleep, anxiety, mood, and various aspects of behavior. In the pineal gland, serotonin is converted to N-acetylserotonin and then ultimately to melatonin. Many health food and nutrition stores also sell tryptophan and 5-HTP as a way for people to boost their levels of serotonin and melatonin. However, whether these supplements actually boost levels of serotonin or melatonin to a significant degree is a subject of debate among scientists.

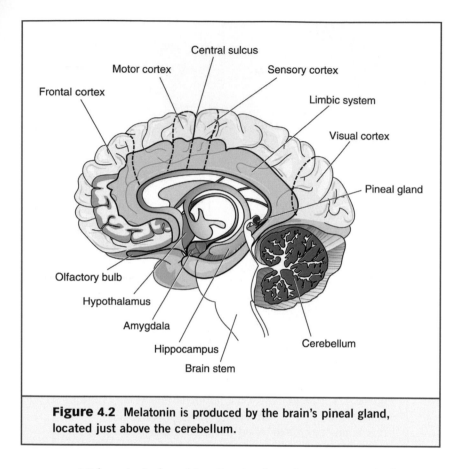

Figure 4.2 Melatonin is produced by the brain's pineal gland, located just above the cerebellum.

Melatonin is found in all animals and even some single-celled organisms. Melatonin production by the pineal gland is low during the day and then increases at night, suggesting that it helps to promote sleep. However, in nocturnal (active at night) animals like rodents and raccoons, melatonin production in the pineal gland is still increased at night and low during the day. So, melatonin may promote sleep in most animals, but in nocturnal animals it may serve some other function, such as promoting wakefulness or reproduction.

In humans, at dusk when the sun is setting and the amount of light entering the eyes decreases, brain regions that receive information from the eyes send signals to the pineal

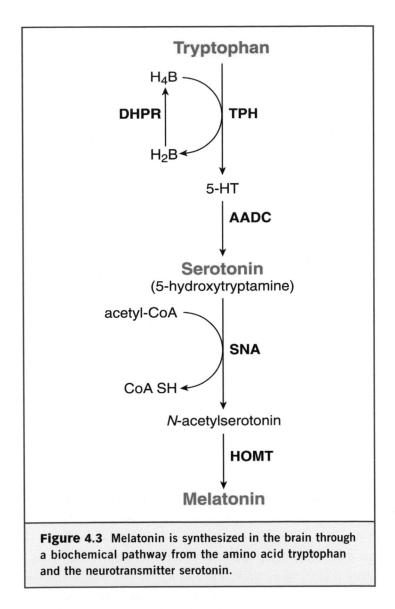

Figure 4.3 Melatonin is synthesized in the brain through a biochemical pathway from the amino acid tryptophan and the neurotransmitter serotonin.

gland to increase the production and release of melatonin (see Figure 4.4). In the morning, when the sun rises and increased sunlight is received by the eyes, these brain regions then send signals to the pineal gland to reduce melatonin synthesis and its release into the bloodstream.

EFFECTS ON SLEEP, BIOLOGICAL RHYTHMS, AND JET LAG

Since melatonin production and secretion from the pineal gland starts to increase in the evening and peaks in the middle of the night, researchers speculate that melatonin promotes sleep. Many studies of the effects of melatonin on sleep in humans have been conducted, but conclusions have been hard to draw since many factors vary between each individual study, such as the dose of melatonin (doses from 0.1 mg to 2,500 mg have been used) and, perhaps more important, time of day of administration (see box on pages 58–59). Overall, the consensus is that melatonin appears to promote sleep only if given when endogenous levels of melatonin (i.e., levels produced by the pineal gland, not a melatonin pill) in the blood are very low (during the day). This is because at night, melatonin secretion is high (refer to Figure 4.4) and it is very difficult to boost those levels any higher by taking a pill containing even high concentrations of melatonin. Thus, melatonin may not be a very effective treatment for insomnia since it does not promote sleep when taken at night.

So, if melatonin doesn't help you sleep at night, why take it? Well, there are actually some very good reasons to take melatonin during the day. One reason is to combat jet lag. Suppose, for example, you fly from New York to Paris on a red-eye flight and arrive the next morning—your biological clock is now off by 10 hours (i.e., you crossed 10 time zones on the flight). So, it might be 10:00 A.M. in Paris and everyone is awake and alert, but your body thinks it's midnight and time to go to sleep. If you wanted to use melatonin to help you sleep and get over the jet lag, wait and take the melatonin that night (say at 10:00 P.M.), because this is when your blood level of melatonin would be low because your body thinks its noon back home.

In addition, if you like to plan ahead and want to minimize the jet lag you might experience on an upcoming trip, melatonin can be used to start resetting your biological clock

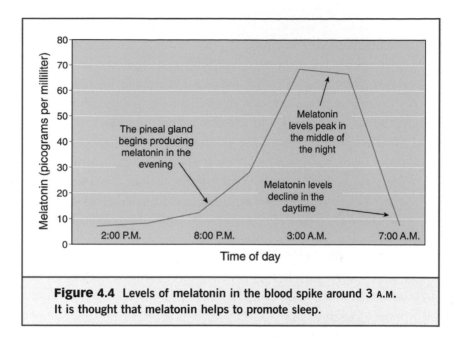

Figure 4.4 Levels of melatonin in the blood spike around 3 A.M. It is thought that melatonin helps to promote sleep.

beforehand. If you are flying eastward (let's say from Portland, Oregon, to London, England), you need to take melatonin at 3:00 P.M. Portland time for several days prior to departure to start resetting your clock, as well as at 3:00 P.M. Portland time on the day of departure. Then, when you arrive in London, you add the number of time zones crossed (i.e., Portland to London is 8 time zones) to 3:00 P.M. (3:00 P.M. + 8 = 11:00 P.M.) and take your melatonin at 11:00 P.M. London time. This will help you sleep the first night and minimize the jet lag you experience. Then, on the next night or two, take melatonin 1 to 2 hours earlier (i.e., 9:00 or 10:00 P.M.) to maximize the ability of melatonin to reset your biological clock.

On the way back, you do the reverse. Take melatonin at 6:00 A.M. London time on the day of departure to reset your clock back to Portland time. When you arrive, you subtract the number of time zones crossed (8) from 6:00 A.M. London time (6:00 A.M. − 8 = 10:00 P.M.) and take melatonin at 10:00 P.M. Portland time the first night back. This will help your body reset its biological clock to your normal pattern of sleeping and waking. However, melatonin is only an aid in resetting your body clock —it actually takes your body approximately one day for each time zone crossed to fully reset your biological clock.

Another reason to take melatonin during the day is if you are a shift worker and your schedule rotates every week or so. For example, Lisa worked as a receptionist at a hospital emergency room. As we all know, emergency rooms don't close for the night and must always have people on staff. Lisa's work schedule was to work 9:30 P.M. to 7:30 A.M. for seven nights and then have seven days off. Of course, during her seven days off

THE SCIENCE OF BIOLOGICAL RHYTHMS

The study of biological rhythms is called **chronobiology**. As discussed in Chapter 1, sleep is a biological rhythm since it takes place at roughly the same time every day. We have many other biological rhythms as well: our hormones rise and fall at regular times throughout the day, as does our body temperature, blood pressure, and even our mental abilities. All animals have similar biological rhythms, although nocturnal animals are on opposite schedules from diurnal creatures like humans. Even some plants have biological rhythms, opening and closing their flower petals in the morning and evening.

In the last two decades, medical science has taken an interest in how some drugs may work more efficiently at certain times of the day. This field, known as chronophar- macology or chronotherapy, is based on the fact that some drugs, whether they are medications designed to help you sleep better, relieve symptoms of psychiatric disorders, fight cancer, or lower blood pressure, actually work better when taken at regular and specific times of the day. Drugs that have these biological timing properties are called chronobiotics or chronotherapeutics.

every other week, Lisa would try to sleep during the day to stay on schedule; but we all know that life makes it hard to sleep during the day. So, Lisa tried taking melatonin at her usual bedtime (10:00 A.M.) during both her weeks on and off work. Remember, just like nocturnal animals, Lisa's pineal gland still produces the most melatonin at night, despite the fact that she works nights, and produces less melatonin during the day. Since Lisa was taking melatonin at a time when her body's own melatonin levels were low, the melatonin pills helped her sleep better during the day and kept her biological clock set for the night shift.

THE SCIENCE OF BIOLOGICAL RHYTHMS (cont.)

For example, a recent study by anesthesiologists in France showed that the narcotic pain reliever sufentanil was more effective in relieving pain during childbirth if the drug was given around noon or midnight and less effective at other times of the day, even though the same dose was given at all times.[5] Findings like these show that, like sleep, our response to certain medications is under the control of biological rhythms. Since chronopharmacology has only been around for a few years, many more studies are needed to determine the most effective times of the day to administer specific drugs.

Drugs that help you sleep are also considered chronobiotics. If you normally sleep from 11:00 P.M. to 7:00 A.M. and were to take an OTC sleeping pill like Nytol at 2:00 P.M., it might make you a little drowsy, but it would be hard to fall asleep since your body's internal clock is usually telling you to be awake at that time. However, if you took it at 10:30 P.M., the drowsiness produced by the sleeping pill should help you fall asleep for the night, because this is around the normal time you go to sleep.

IS MELATONIN SAFE?

Doses of melatonin as low as 3 mg (if given during the day) can produce increases in blood levels of melatonin that are 50 times higher than normal levels. Thus, "megadose" pills offered by some health food stores may cause melatonin concentrations that are vastly in excess of what is needed to affect sleep or biological rhythms. Melatonin is metabolized by the liver fairly quickly, so that half of the ingested melatonin is eliminated from the body within an hour of taking it, and an entire 3 mg dose is eliminated in 6 to 10 hours.

Studies in both animals and humans indicate that taking melatonin is extremely safe, with very few people reporting any side effects. However, possible side effects of taking it for months or years have not been examined. Most melatonin available over-the-counter is chemically synthesized and not extracted from the pineal gland of animals. Several pharmaceutical companies are currently developing melatonin analogues (closely related molecules that act just like melatonin) for the potential treatment of jet lag and to help shift workers better adapt to their schedules.

5

Over-the-Counter Stimulants

Stimulants are most often used to counteract sleepiness, increase energy levels, and aid weight loss. We might use stimulants to overcome sleepiness in order to study for exams or for simply staying awake in class or at work. These drugs are part of our daily lives, whether we take them in the form coffee from Starbucks®, carbonated beverages or chocolate candy bars, diet pills, or medications for pain, allergies, and the common cold (Figure 5.1). Stimulants increase the activity of the central nervous system to increase alertness, and they also act in other parts of the body to increase heart and breathing rates, blood pressure, muscle tension, urination, perspiration, dilation of the airways, and blood supply to the brain and skeletal muscles.

Despite their ability to keep us awake, stimulants can produce unwanted side effects, such as anxiety, muscle tremor (the "shakes"), sweating, hyperthermia, insomnia, and headaches, especially when taken in larger than recommended quantities. In addition, some stimulants are addictive when taken repeatedly, and when their use is stopped suddenly, withdrawal symptoms can occur that include depression, fatigue, irritability, nausea, and headaches.

The main classes of over-the-counter stimulants contain caffeine, ephedrine/pseudoephedrine, or herbal varieties of stimulants. Each of these will be discussed in this chapter.

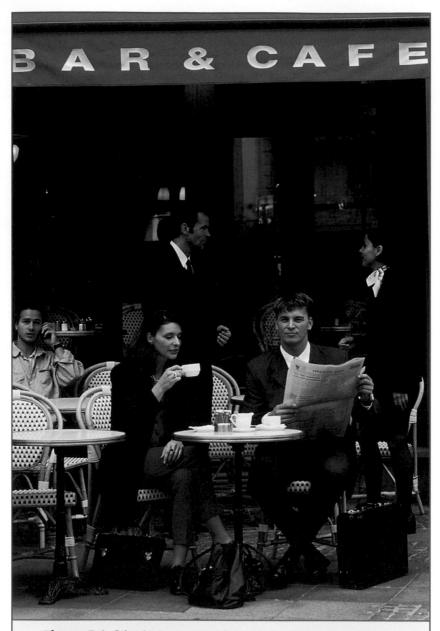

Figure 5.1 Stimulants are most often used to counteract sleepiness, whether taken in the form of coffee, carbonated beverages, candy bars, diet pills, or medications.

CAFFEINE

Caffeine is the most widely used OTC stimulant in the United States. This is a direct result of the fact that, in recent decades, our society has become "24/7" and constantly on the go. As a result, there is a vastly increased number and variety of caffeine-containing coffees, teas, cola beverages, and "energy drinks" such as Red Bull® (Table 5.1). However, in addition to being a common ingredient in such beverages, caffeine is the sole active ingredient in OTC stimulants such as Nodoz®, Caffedrine®, Enerjets®, Vivarin®, Stimerall®, Quick Lift®, Blue Alert®, and Bolt Magnum®. Such caffeine pills contain higher levels of caffeine than ordinary caffeine-containing beverages.

Table 5.1. Comparison of Caffeine Levels

SOURCE	AMOUNT OF CAFFEINE
Cola	30–60 mg per 12 ounces
Coffee, brewed	40–180 mg per cup
Coffee, instant	30–120 mg per cup
Tea	20–110 mg per cup
Sweet chocolate	20 mg per ounce
Milk chocolate	6 mg per ounce
Hot cocoa	2–8 mg per 6 ounces
Caffeine pill	200 mg per pill

Caffeine is also present in some pain relievers, such as Anacin®, Excedrin®, and Midol®, and cold remedies, such as Dristan® and Triaminicin®.

Caffeine has the effect of promoting wakefulness while delaying the onset of sleep. If taken only on occasion, caffeine pills are generally safe to use as a way to combat sleepiness. However, if taken regularly, tolerance can develop (i.e., the need for increasing doses to obtain the same effect), which often leads to caffeine addiction. In addition, taking caffeine regularly can increase the likelihood of experiencing insomnia, anxiety, nervousness, irritability, headaches, and stomach problems, especially if consuming caffeine is stopped suddenly. Some tips for avoiding caffeine addiction are:

- Limit your intake to 200–300 mg per day.

- Drink herbal teas or decaffeinated drinks.

- Get regular exercise instead of relying on caffeine pills for your energy.

- Eat regular meals.

- Do not consume caffeine after 4 P.M.

In addition to being a stimulant, caffeine also has many effects outside of the nervous system. Caffeine is a cardio-vascular stimulant, causing the heart rate to increase while constricting blood vessels, both of which can cause increases in blood pressure. Caffeine is also a diuretic (i.e., it increases urination), so it can sometimes cause dehydration and low calcium levels. If taken during pregnancy, the amount of caffeine should be limited to 300 mg per day, as birth problems have been reported in pregnant women who consume more than this amount.

Caffeine acts in the brain by blocking receptors for the neurotransmitter adenosine. Normally, adenosine helps to calm nerve cells and promote sleep, but when the receptors for adenosine are blocked by caffeine, the result is the opposite: an increase in the activity of the nervous system and thus increased alertness.

Although rare, it is possible to overdose on caffeine. In the late 1990s, a North Carolina community college student swallowed almost 90 caffeine pills (equivalent to about 250 cups of coffee) and later died as a result.

EPHEDRINE AND PSEUDOEPHEDRINE

Ephedrine is a powerful central nervous system stimulant that, up until recently, was commonly found in many diet and weight-loss aids, such as Easy Trim®, Metabolife®, Minithin®, Ripped Fuel®, and Xenadrine®. It is derived from the Chinese herb *ma huang* (also called ephedra), although it is often produced synthetically. Ephedrine suppresses appetite and has also been marketed as a way to increase energy, muscle mass, athletic performance and sexual potency (Figure 5.2a). Because of its stimulant properties, ephedrine has been used by people attempting to stay awake for extended periods of time, such as truck drivers, students studying for exams, and night shift workers.

Although ephedrine has been sold for decades, it has recently been reported that this drug is potentially quite dangerous. Ephedrine use has been linked to numerous heart attacks and strokes (see the box on pages 68–69) and was officially banned by the U.S. Food and Drug Administration (FDA) in February 2004. However, prior to its ban, it was estimated that 12 to 17 million Americans were consuming ephedrine-containing products at an estimated 3 billion doses per year.

A chemical cousin of ephedrine, pseudoephedrine (Figure 5.2b) is found in many allergy and cold medications, such as Sudafed® and Actifed®, and acts to open nasal passages and sinuses to clear nasal congestion. Pseudoephedrine is also a nervous system stimulant—it is much less potent than

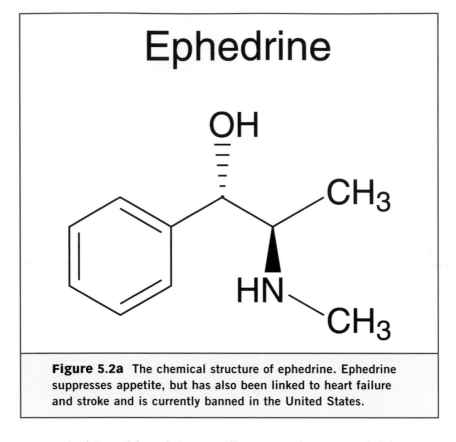

Figure 5.2a The chemical structure of ephedrine. Ephedrine suppresses appetite, but has also been linked to heart failure and stroke and is currently banned in the United States.

ephedrine, although it can still cause restlessness and delay the onset of sleep. In addition, another chemical cousin of ephedrine, called phenylpropanolamine, was used in some cold mediations (Allerest®, Dimetapp®, 4-Way Formula®, and Nyquil®) and weight-loss aids (Acutrim®, Dexatrim®, and Metabolift®). However, phenylpropanolamine was linked to heart problems and strokes, so in 2000 the FDA requested that pharmaceutical manufacturers remove this ingredient from their products.

HERBAL STIMULANTS AND ENERGY BOOSTERS

Nowadays, many gas stations and minimarts sell quick "pick-me-up" stimulant pills that are marketed as "herbal"

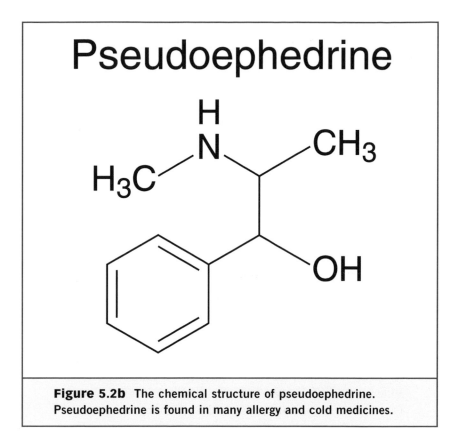

Figure 5.2b The chemical structure of pseudoephedrine. Pseudoephedrine is found in many allergy and cold medicines.

or "natural." However, these "herbal" stimulants actually contain the same stimulants—caffeine, ephedrine, or pseudo-ephedrine—but in a natural herbal form. For example, the Chinese herb *ma huang* contains ephedra, which is ephedrine found in its natural source, an herbal plant. However, although the FDA has banned ephedrine, ephedra in its herbal form can still be found in some products, although it remains on the FDA's watchlist of potentially dangerous drugs.

Other herbal stimulants include guarana or kola, which are natural sources of caffeine, just like the coffee bean. There are many such concoctions of caffeine or ephedra on the market, or recently taken off the market (Table 5.2).

(continued on page 72)

DANGERS OF EPHEDRINE

Ephedrine was a popular ingredient in many diet pills and muscle and energy boosters for decades. Ephedrine-based products were marketed to teenagers and young adults as having the ability to produce euphoria (feelings of pleasure) and increased sexual sensations, energy, and alertness. However, over the last decade, scientists have linked ephedrine use to numerous heart attacks, strokes, and deaths.

Concerns about the safety of ephedrine-containing products date back to 1994, when the FDA noticed an increase in the number of health problems associated with the use of ephedrine, including chest pain, headaches, increased blood pressure, heart attack, hepatitis (inflammation of the liver), stroke, seizures, and sometimes death. In 2001, the National Football League banned the use of ephedrine by professional football players. The National Collegiate Athletic Association (NCAA) and Olympic committees have also banned the use of ephedrine by their athletes. In February 2004, ephedrine was finally banned by the FDA from being sold in the United States. To date, at least 100 deaths have been attributed to ephedrine use in the U.S. alone. Here are some examples of the potentially deadly effects of ephedrine:

- A 19-year-old college student, working late nights at a gas station, began taking OTC ephedrine pills to help him stay awake at work. After taking a total of four pills in a 24-hour period, he collapsed and died while pumping gas. An autopsy revealed that the student suffered a massive heart attack triggered by ephedrine toxicity.

- A 17-year-old high school football player started to take ephedrine to enhance his performance and increase his energy levels during football games.

One night after going to bed, he suffered a major heart attack and died. An autopsy revealed that the heart attack was a result of ephedrine, although he never exceeded the recommended dosage.

- A 16-year-old high school student started taking ephedrine in an attempt to lose weight. Soon after taking the pills, she experienceed heart palpitations (very strong heart beats) and collapsed during a sporting event. Fortunately, she survived, but she had to be treated for years for an irregular heartbeat brought on by the ephedrine pills.

- In August 2004, a jury awarded $4.1 million in damages against a sports nutrition store that sold products containing ephedrine. The lawsuit was brought by a man who suffered a massive stroke resulting in brain damage after taking the dietary supplement Dymetadrine Xtreme, which contained ephedra. The man must now use a wheelchair or walker to move around and has trouble with speech and double vision.

- Ephedrine is now banned at U.S. military bases worldwide after two dozen soldiers died from taking ephedrine to boost energy levels and combat sleepiness.

Now that ephedrine-based OTC pills are banned, many manufacturers of the drug are seeking to find alternative ingredients that may produce the same stimulant effects. So, many nutrition products are often labeled as "ephedrine free." However, the potential health hazards of such replacement ingredients have not been fully studied by the FDA.

In February 2003, Baltimore Orioles pitcher Steve Bechler, 23, was in spring training in Florida and started to complain of fatigue and an inability to run as much as he could previously. Then, on February 17, Bechler collapsed from apparent heat stroke and later died (Figure 5.3). It turned out that Bechler had been taking the diet supplement Xenadrine, which contains ephedrine, in an attempt to lose weight. Doctors ruled that the official cause of death was heat stroke—Bechler's core body temperature was 106°F at the time he was removed from the practice field. While doctors speculate that ephedrine played a role in the death of the promising young baseball player, it is likely that pre-existing health problems and other factors also contributed to Bechler's death. Such factors and health problems included:

- A prior history of heat illness episodes while in high school.

- A history of high blood pressure and liver problems.

- Taking ephedrine on an empty stomach (he had not eaten solid food for at least 24 hours in an apparent attempt to lose weight).

- He was overweight.

- He was exercising in high temperatures.

Thus, ephedrine can apparently interact with other health factors that may increase the hazards of using it as a stimulant. Despite this, Bechler's widow has filed a $600 million lawsuit against the manufacturers of Xenadrine.

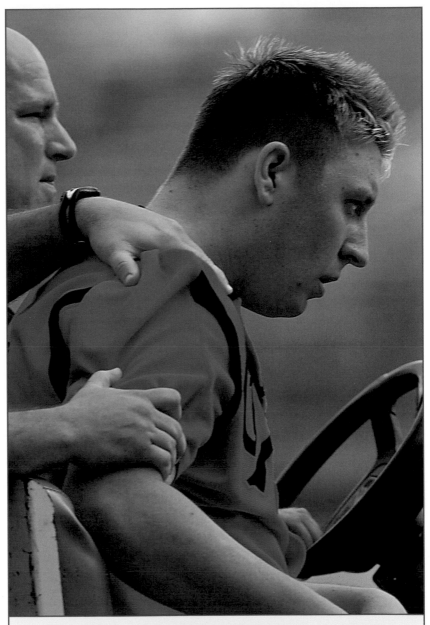

Figure 5.3 The death of Baltimore Orioles pitcher Steve Bechler, 23, has been linked to the use of ephedrine-containing diet supplements. Bechler, seen here, is being helped off the field.

Table 5.2 Common Herbal Stimulants

BRAND NAME	HERBAL INGREDIENT	ACTIVE INGREDIENT
Kicker Chinese Herbs	*ma huang*	ephedra
Ultra Energy Now	*ma huang* guarana extract kola	ephedra caffeine
Gin Zing™	*ma huang* guarana	ephedra caffeine
Mega BLAST High	*ma huang*	ephedra
Energy Formula	gota kola	caffeine
Super PEP Extra Strength	kola nut gota kola guarana	caffeine caffeine caffeine
Super Ener-Max	*ma huang* green tea extract kola nut	ephedra caffeine caffeine

(continued from page 67)

Such herbal stimulants are particularly dangerous to teenagers for a variety of reasons:

- Teens are likely to be persuaded by marketing claims.

- Teens (especially girls) are at a very high risk for anorexia or bulimia and the overuse of stimulants such as weight-loss aids.

- The terms *herbal* or *natural* can lead to a false sense of security.

- Teens often believe in the attitude that taking more than the recommended dose is not harmful.

- There are no legal controls on the sale, consumption, or distribution of herbal stimulants.

6

Prescription Sleep Aids and Stimulants

Most over-the-counter sleep aids are relatively mild and can be used effectively to treat temporary sleeping problems such as insomnia. However, when insomnia is persistent and results in sleepiness during the day that disrupts your ability to perform at work or stay awake in class, it may be necessary to obtain a doctor's prescription for a more potent sleep aid. Prescription sleep aids are often referred to as "hypnotics" and they decrease the time it takes to fall asleep and keep you asleep longer.

There are also some cases when a doctor's prescription is needed to obtain a stimulant in order to keep the person awake. Such cases include people with narcolepsy, who are extremely sleepy much of the day, and people who have jobs that require prolonged periods of wakefulness, such as soldiers in the military, long-haul truck drivers, and people who work night shifts or rotating shift-work schedules.

BARBITURATES

Barbiturate drugs like pentobarbital (Nembutal®), secobarbital (Seconal®), amobarbital (Amytal®), and phenobarbital are extremely potent sedatives that induce sleep, mostly non-REM sleep. However, barbiturates actually decrease the amount of REM sleep a person gets. Thus, if a person took a barbiturate as a sleep aid nightly for a week, the total amount of REM sleep would be significantly less than if he or she was not taking the drug. Then, when the person stopped taking the barbiturate, he or she would experience a severe "REM rebound," or dramatic increase in REM sleep. Such a rebound can often lead to nightmares in people undergoing barbiturate withdrawal.

Barbiturates have many other unwanted side effects: they are addicting, they produce tolerance (less of an effect observed over time after repeatedly taking the medication), they slow breathing and have the potential to cause overdoses and death, and they interfere with the body's ability to metabolize other drugs, causing unpredictable drug interactions. For decades throughout the early- to mid-twentieth century, barbiturates were commonly used as prescription sleep aids. However, in 1979, the Institute of Medicine issued a report stating that the risks of using barbiturates far outweighed their benefits for treating insomnia. Some barbiturates were even taken off the market because of the risks they posed. Today, prescribing barbiturates for sleep problems is very rare and considered obsolete.

BENZODIAZEPINES

In the 1960s and 1970s, scientists developed a newer class of drugs called benzodiazepines, which appeared to be safer and more effective sleep aids than barbiturates. One of the first benzodiazepines to be developed was diazepam (Valium), which is still commonly prescribed today for the treatment of anxiety.

Like barbiturates, benzodiazepines reduce the activity of the nervous system. They do this by acting on the type-A GABA (or $GABA_A$) receptor, which is the protein that the neurotransmitter GABA activates when it is secreted by one nerve cell onto another (refer back to Chapter 1 for an overview of how nerve cells communicate). When this receptor binds GABA, nerve cells become less active. Thus, like GABA, benzodiazepines "deactivate" nerve cells.

There are many kinds of benzodiazepines that differ slightly in their chemical structure. They also differ in how long it takes the body to get rid of them once they are ingested.

The length of time it takes for the body to metabolize or eliminate half of the drug taken is called its **half-life**. For example, if you took 10 mg of a benzodiazepine that has a half-life of four hours, then four hours after you took the drug, 5 mg of it would remain in your system. In another four hours, 2.5 mg would remain, four hours later only 1.25 mg would remain, and so on, until the drug is completely eliminated from the body. The half-life is an important factor when a doctor determines which benzodiazepine to prescribe, based on the needs of the patient. For example, Valium has a half-life of approximately 30 hours, so it stays in the body for a long time. This is good for people who suffer from anxiety, since having the drug wear off more quickly would mean taking pills more often. However, when benzodiazepines are used to treat trouble falling asleep, shorter half-lives (an hour or two) are preferable, because if the drug remained in the body in significant quantities after 8 hours of sleep, the person would remain sleepy during the next day. But if a person has trouble staying asleep throughout the night, a benzodiazepine with a longer half-life might be better suited for them. Table 6.1 shows common benzodiazepines used as sleep aids, with their usual dose and half-life.

Compared to barbiturates, benzodiazepines are relatively safe medications that produce little tolerance and suppression of REM sleep, and benzodiazepine overdoses are much less common. However, benzodiazepines are not without unwanted side effects. As mentioned above, longer-acting benzodiazepines can produce residual drowsiness, grogginess, and weakness the next day (benzodiazepines are also muscle relaxants). Benzodiazepines can produce rebound insomnia, in which the person experiences significant insomnia after he or she stops taking the medication. This is particularly true with benzodiazepines that have short half-lives. To avoid this, the patient should never stop "cold turkey;" rather, the dosage should be slowly tapered off over several days to a week.

Table 6.1 Common Benzodiazepines Used as Sleep Aids

DRUG	BRAND NAME	USUAL DOSE	APPROXIMATE HALF-LIFE
Flurazepam	Dalmane®	15–30 mg	40–250 hours*
Quazepam	Doral®	7.5–15 mg	40–250 hours*
Clonazepam	Klonopin	0.5–3.0 mg	18–50 hours
Estazolam	ProSom®	1–2 mg	10–24 hours*
Temazepam	Restoril®	7.5–15 mg	8–22 hours
Midazolam	Versed®	7.5–15 mg	1–3 hours
Triazolam	Halcion	0.125–0.250 mg	1–3 hours

* Note: Flurazepam, quazepam, and estazolam are not particularly effective sleep aids on their own, but they are metabolized by the body into molecules that are effective sleep aids and also extremely long-acting.

In addition, some benzodiazepines cause dizziness, confusion, clumsiness and falling, and memory loss when the drug levels in the body are at their highest. This can be a problem if you are awakened in the middle of the night by a fire alarm, a crying baby that needs to be fed, or some other reason. Also, there are potential serious interactions of benzodiazepines with alcohol—if a person drinks alcohol after taking a benzodiazepine, extreme sedation can result. Benzodiazepines can also worsen the symptoms of sleep apnea (see Chapter 2). Finally, benzodiazepines are not meant to be taken for long periods of time (more than 4 weeks), as this can potentially lead to dependence or addiction to these drugs.

More recently, several drugs have been developed that are not classified as benzodiazepines because their chemical structure is slightly different from benzodiazepines (see Figure 6.1). These drugs are extremely popular and are currently the most widely prescribed sleep aids, as shown in Table 6.2.

LAWSUITS: "THE DRUG MADE ME DO IT"

In recent years, many lawsuits have been brought against pharmaceutical manufacturers, claiming that drugs intended to treat psychiatric conditions, such as depression, anxiety, and even insomnia, cause people to become aggressive, violent, or suicidal. Over 150 lawsuits have been brought against Eli Lilly & Company, the manufacturer of the antidepressant Prozac, claiming that the drug caused some patients to commit murder or suicide after taking the drug. Recently a teenager in South Carolina was charged with murdering his grandparents, and the boy's defense was that an adverse reaction to an antidepressant caused his violent behavior.

In many people with psychiatric disorders such as severe depression, thoughts of aggression and suicide are common. There is a great deal of debate as to whether the person experiences such thoughts as a result of the medication or the disorder itself. In fact, it may be almost impossible to determine if it is the psychiatric disorder or the medication designed to treat it that causes the violent thoughts and behaviors.

Since these newer drugs have such short half-lives, they rarely result in "hang-over" effects and grogginess the next morning. Ambien and Sonata are usually prescribed for people having trouble falling asleep, and Lunesta® and Imovane® are prescribed for people who have trouble staying asleep. These medications are quite safe and they also have virtually no suppression of REM sleep, and they are less likely to cause tolerance, addiction, and withdrawal. However, these medications still have potentially adverse effects on sleep apnea and significant interaction with alcohol.

LAWSUITS: "THE DRUG MADE ME DO IT" (cont.)

With regard to prescription sleep aids, approximately 100 lawsuits have been brought against the Upjohn Company, the manufacturer of the benzodiazepine Halcion, claiming that the medication causes patients to suffer psychiatric reactions, such as paranoia, suidical thinking, aggression, and bizarre behavior. In 1991, Britain banned the sale of Halcion, and the Upjohn Company strengthened its warning labels on Halcion package inserts in the United States and also cut the recommended dosages in half. They also added recommendations that the drug not be taken if the patient is currently taking an antidepressant medication.

So, if a person taking a psychiatric medication commits a crime, who is responsible—the patient taking the medication, the doctor who prescribes it, the pharmacy that sells the drug, or the company that manufactures it? In 1992, a jury found William Freeman, a former assistant police chief in Texas who was taking Halcion, guilty of murdering his friend. But the jury divided up the blame, saying that Freeman was 50% responsible, the doctor 30% responsible, and the Upjohn Company 20% responsible. However, the verdict was later appealed and overturned.[6]

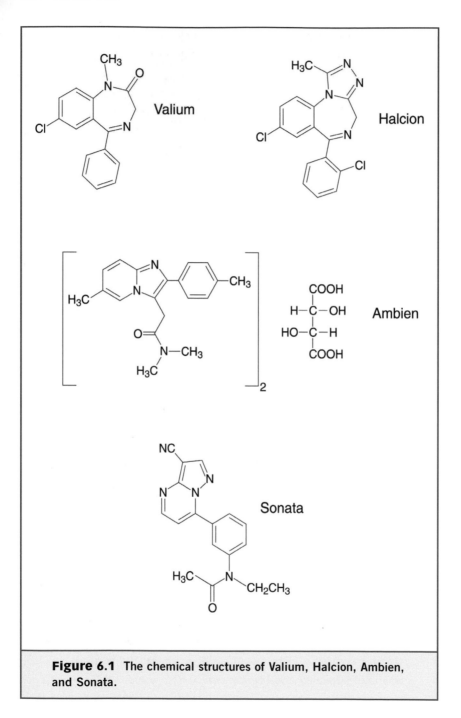

Figure 6.1 The chemical structures of Valium, Halcion, Ambien, and Sonata.

Table 6.2 Non-Benzodiazepine Medications Used as Sleep Aids

DRUG	BRAND NAME	USUAL DOSE	APPROXIMATE HALF-LIFE
Zolpidem	Ambien	5–10 mg	2.5 hours
Zaleplon	Sonata	5–20 mg	1 hour
Zopiclone	Imovane	5.0–7.5 mg	5 hours
Eszopiclone	Lunesta	1–3 mg	6 hours

PRESCRIPTION STIMULANTS

Although most of this chapter has focused on prescription sleep aids, there are a few prescription medications available to help you stay awake. The most commonly used OTC stimulant is caffeine. However, people with the sleep disorder narcolepsy are very sleepy during the day (no matter how much sleep they get) and often require prescription stimulants to alleviate their sleepiness. Stimulants are also prescribed for the treatment of attention deficit/hyperactivity disorder (ADHD, sometimes called ADD), asthma, and obesity.

Stimulants increase the overall activity of the nervous system by boosting the release of various neurotransmitters such as dopamine, norepinephrine, and glutamate. The result is increased alertness, attention, and energy. Unfortunately, prescription stimulants can be highly addictive and cause cardiovascular side effects (increased heart rate, blood pressure, and irregular heart rate) as well as respiratory side effects (dilated airways and increased breathing rate). Taking stimulants repeatedly and in excessive doses can

Amy was having trouble sleeping, so she asked her doctor for a sleeping pill. Her doctor felt that Amy was suffering from a brief bout of insomnia and prescribed her a three-day supply of a popular sleeping pill. The first night, she took the pill at 9:15 P.M., about 45 minutes before her normal bedtime, and fell asleep by about 9:45 P.M. Then, at 10:30 P.M., Amy's friend called her, wanting to talk about troubles she was having with her boyfriend. The phone woke up Amy and she instinctively answered it, but she soon realized that she felt strange. She was a little dizzy and confused and had a hard time focusing on the conversation with her friend. Her mind drifted as she tried to stay awake, and she often found herself responding to her friend by saying, "Ummm . . . what?" Finally, Amy told her friend that she had just taken a sleeping pill and would have to talk to her the next day. Amy simply couldn't maintain the conversation.

Dizziness and the inability to concentrate are common side effects that one might experience if awakened within a few hours of taking a prescription sleep aid. In Amy's case, the result was just a postponed conversation. However, imagine if you were awakened to the sound of a smoke alarm and had to get up, get dressed, and run outside of a burning house, all the while being confused as to what was going on and how to get out of the house. In cases like this, one would surely rather have insomnia than be trapped inside of a burning building.

Sleeping pills can be a blessing to someone who is suffering from insomnia, but there are always unforeseeable events. This is why prescription sleep aids should only be taken under the orders of a doctor, and only if the insomnia has proven untreatable with OTC sleep aids or other non-prescription methods.

cause paranoia, hostility, and, in extreme cases, seizures, heart failure, dangerously high body temperatures, and even death. These potentially harmful side effects are the reason that doctors prescribe stimulants only when medically necessary, as in the case of narcolepsy. A doctor will not usually prescribe a stimulant to help you stay awake to study for exams. However, a recent study indicated that as many as 7% of college students take prescription stimulants (prescribed to treat a medical condition) for non-medical purposes, such as staying up late to study or socialize.[7] In addition, some teenagers who use these medications have been caught illegally giving away or selling their medications to fellow students to experiments with.[8]

Table 6.3 Commonly Prescribed Stimulants

DRUG	BRAND NAME	APPROXIMATE HALF-LIFE
methylphenidate	Ritalin	2–3 hours
pemoline	Cylert	10–14 hours
dextroamphetamine	Dexedrine	10–13 hours
modafinil	ProVigil	12–15 hours

Some of these drugs, such as Dexedrine, are derivatives of the illegal stimulant amphetamine. Some drugs, such as Adderall®, are also used to treat narcolepsy and ADHD and actually contain a mixture of dextroamphetamine and amphetamine.

As an aside, in March of 2005, Abbott Laboratories, the maker of Cylert®, decided to take its drug off the U.S. market because of increasing concerns about it causing liver problems. Cylert® had been available in the United States for 30 years for the treatment of ADHD and narcolepsy. However, the generic form of Cylert® (pemoline) is still available.

7

Other Drugs and Medications

In previous chapters, we examined drugs specifically intended to keep you awake (such as caffeine) and drugs that are specifically intended to help you sleep (such as benzodiazepines). There are, however, many medications that are taken for the purpose of treating other medical conditions—allergies, high blood pressure, epilepsy, obesity, chronic pain, and psychiatric disorders such as schizophrenia and depression—that also can affect your sleep. In addition, addictive drugs such as alcohol, nicotine, and cocaine have strong effects on sleep.

ANTIHISTAMINES

As mentioned in Chapter 3, antihistamines are the main active ingredients in OTC sleeping pills since they are moderately effective in causing drowsiness. However, antihistamines are also widely used for the treatment of allergies because they block the effects of histamine, which is released by immune cells to cause sneezing, runny nose, and itchy eyes. Since the histamine molecule released by immune cells outside the nervous system is the same one inside the nervous system that regulates sleeping and waking, antihistamines that are designed to fight allergies also can cause drowsiness. So, antihistamines should not be taken prior to driving a car or operating dangerous machinery.

WEIGHT-LOSS DRUGS

Most weight-loss drugs are actually central nervous system stimulants. These stimulants, such as phentermine (an ingredient in the now banned weight-loss drug PhenFen) and Mazindol, suppress appetite and cause nerve cells to release the neurotransmitters dopamine, norephinephrine, and serotonin. Although these drugs are not as potent as stimulants like amphetamine, they do have the ability to promote wakefulness. As a result, people taking weight-loss drugs often experience insomnia as a side effect, particularly if the drug is taken in the evening.

BLOOD PRESSURE AND HEART MEDICATIONS

Medications that are used to treat high blood pressure generally act by relaxing the smooth muscle walls of the arteries, causing them to dilate and reduce blood pressure. They accomplish this by blocking the activity of adrenergic receptors, proteins that are normally activated by the neurotransmitters norepinephrine and epinephrine. There are several types of adrenergic receptors, one of which is called the beta adrenergic receptor (thus medications that inhibit the activity of this receptor are called "beta blockers"). Common beta blockers include propranolol (Inderal®), atenolol (Tenormin®) acebutolol (Sectral®), pindolol (Visken®), bisoprolol (Cardicor®), carvedilol (Eucardic®), and metoprolol (Betaloc®). Beta blockers can also correct heart beat irregularities (arrhythmias) and reduce chest pain (angina). Sleep disturbances are often reported by people taking this type of medication, with daytime drowsiness, fragmented sleep (sleep with frequent awakenings), and increased nightmares the most common complaints. This is believed to result from interference by these drugs with the beta adrenergic receptors in the brain, which play an important role in the regulation of sleep and dreaming.

Other types of blood pressure medications, such as clonidine, act by stimulating alpha adrenergic receptors, which have the same effect in reducing blood pressure as beta blockers. The most common side effect of clonidine is sedation and drowsiness.

EPILEPSY MEDICATIONS

Epilepsy is a neurological disorder caused by severe over-activity of the nervous system, which results in convulsions and seizures (moderate to violent shaking, loss of control of the arms and limbs, and often a loss of consciousness). Drugs that are designed to treat epilepsy are called anti-epileptics or anticonvulsants. These drugs act by decreasing the overall activity of the nervous system, usually by increasing the activity of the $GABA_A$ receptor (see Chapter 6) or by some related mechanism. Benzodiazepines are moderately effective at reducing seizures, but other more potent anticonvulsant medications include phenytoin (Dilantin®), valproate (Depakote®), topiramate (Topamax®), tiagabine (Gabitril®), carbamazepine (Tegretol®, Epitol®), gabapentin (Neurontin®), and lamotrigine (Lamictal®). Since these medications reduce the overall activity of the nervous system, sedation and drowsiness are common side effects.

ANTIDEPRESSANTS

Depression, especially severe depression, is often accompanied by sleep disturbances, such as difficulty falling asleep, fragmented sleep (frequent awakenings), and early morning awakenings. In addition, the structure of a person's sleep may be altered in depression, such as decreased total non-REM sleep and a reduction in the time it takes to enter the first REM period of the night. Antidepressant drugs often bring immediate relief for these sleep problems, but improvement in the depression may not occur until after several weeks of taking the drug.

Most of the newer antidepressant medications such as fluoxetine (Prozac), fluvoxamine (Luvox®), paroxetine (Paxil), sertraline (Zoloft), and citalopram (Celexa), act by reducing the ability of nerve cells to reabsorb and reuse the neuro-transmitter serotonin after it has been released. This results in extra amounts of serotonin that can bind to and alter the function of neighboring nerve cells. Serotonin is found in many regions of the brain that control sleep and, as a result, antidepressants can alter sleep significantly. Common side effects of antidepressant medications are sedation and drowsiness, although some people actually feel more energetic after taking an antidepressant (which may be due to a partial relief of the depression symptoms).

As mentioned in Chapter 2, another side effect of these newer types of antidepressants is that they can cause people to show signs of REM behavior disorder, which is characterized by periodic moments of acting out dreams. Rather than having the person stop taking the antidepressant altogether to avoid this, many times a doctor will prescribe a benzodiazepine such as clonazepam (Klonopin) that helps to suppress the REM behavior disorder symptoms.

MEDICATIONS FOR SCHIZOPHRENIA

Schizophrenia is a devastating mental disorder characterized by abnormal thinking, psychosis (delusions, paranoia, hearing voices), lack of emotion, and loss of function in one's school or workplace. The bizarre thought patterns of schizophrenics often resemble that of dream content, and in fact it was once hypothesized that people with schizophrenia suffered from "intrusions" of REM sleep into wakefulness, much like that seen in people with narcolepsy. However, most scientific evidence suggests that this is not the case.

Schizophrenia is usually treated with a class of medications called antipsychotics, or neuroleptics, that act to reduce the activity of the neurotransmitter dopamine, which may be overactive in the brains of schizophrenics. Commonly used antipsychotic medications include risperidone (Risperdal®), haloperidol (Haldol®), olanzapine (Zyprexa®), quetiapine (Seroquel®), clozapine (Clozaril®), aripiprazole (Abilify®), and ziprasidone (Geodon®). Many of these drugs have the side effect of sedation and drowsiness, primarily because it is thought that dopamine is necessary for promoting wakefulness, and therefore blocking the activity of dopamine would produce the opposite effect.

PAIN MEDICATIONS

Although OTC pain medications, for the most part, do not significantly alter sleep, prescription pain medications, including opiates like morphine and Demerol, do have effects on sleep. Most opiate painkillers are sedating and cause drowsiness, but once the person is actually asleep they can reduce the amount of time spent in REM sleep. In fact, if a person takes an opiate pain reliever for an extended period of time, he or she can experience "REM rebound" after stopping the medication, since REM sleep is suppressed when the person is taking the drug. Opiate pain relievers also suppress breathing and, thus, if taken by a person with sleep apnea (see Chapter 2), may make their condition significantly worse.

ALCOHOL, NICOTINE, AND OTHER ADDICTIVE DRUGS

Although many of alcohol's effects depend on an individual's sensitivity to it, one to two drinks of alcohol do not really alter a person's sleep to a significant degree. In fact, this amount of alcohol may cause a person to become slightly hyperactive. However, larger amounts of alcohol cause drowsiness and decrease the amount of time it takes to fall asleep. But, once the "drunk" person is asleep, their sleep patterns become very fragmented. REM sleep is initially suppressed in the first part of the night, but it increases in the latter half of the night.

Alcohol, particularly as it is being processed by the body, also causes frequent awakenings, although the person may not actually remember them. In addition, a person who drinks alcohol regularly may experience REM rebound during withdrawal, much the way a person would after taking an opiate pain reliever. Alcohol is a muscle relaxant and also suppresses breathing during sleep, so people who have sleep apnea often find that their disorder is made significantly worse by drinking alcohol. Alcohol can also cause short episodes of sleep apnea in people who otherwise do not have the disorder.

Nicotine, the addictive ingredient of tobacco and cigarettes, does not alter sleep to a significant degree. However, when a person who is attempting to quit smoking goes through withdrawal, they will likely suffer from difficulty sleeping, irritability, and restlessness. Although nicotine stimulates breathing, it is not particularly effective in treating sleep apnea, especially since it is highly addictive.

Powerful illegal stimulants such as cocaine, amphetamines, MDMA (ecstasy), and methamphetamine produce wakefulness and alertness when the drug levels in the body are at their highest, even when the drug is taken at night. Some drug addicts go on 3 or 4-day drug "binges," taking the drug repeatedly every few hours and not sleeping for days. However, when the drug wears off (or the person runs out of drug supply or money), he or she may "crash" and sleep for long periods of time and also experience signs of depression.

Delta-9-tetrahydrocannabinol (THC), the main active ingredient in marijuana, reduces the amount of time spent in REM sleep, although tolerance to this effect can develop over time and the overall amount of time spent in REM sleep returns to normal levels. However, like people who constantly drink alcohol or take narcotic pain relievers, people who smoke marijuana daily can experience REM rebound after stopping the drug.

Appendix

TIPS FOR GETTING A GOOD NIGHT'S SLEEP

- Avoid smoking or consuming drinks containing caffeine or alcohol late in the afternoon or in the evening. These substances can delay your ability to fall asleep or stay asleep.

- If you have trouble falling asleep, avoid taking naps during the day since they affect your ability to sleep at night.

- Exercise regularly, but do not exercise within one to three hours of your normal bedtime. Exercise increases your body temperature, which makes it more difficult to fall asleep if you have not had enough time to cool down.

- Maintain a regular bedtime and bedtime routine that allows you to unwind and send a signal to your brain that it is time to go to bed.

- Avoid exposure to bright lights (i.e., sun lamps) for one to three hours prior to bedtime, since this can throw off your body's biological clock.

- Avoid using your bed for stimulating activities such as reading, studying, playing computer games, etc. You need to establish an association between being in bed and sleeping. This will help send a signal to your brain that it is time to sleep when you get into bed.

- If you can't fall asleep within 30 minutes of going to bed, don't lie in your bed tossing and turning. Get up, find a quiet relaxing activity to do (such as reading or listening to relaxing music), and when you start to feel sleepy, return to bed.

- During the time you are falling asleep, do not try to solve complex school or personal problems. The best thing that promotes sleep is a trouble-free mind.[9]

Glossary

Antihistamines—Drugs that block the activity of the neurotransmitter histamine, which promotes wakefulness and also causes allergy symptoms.

Atonia—Loss of muscle tone.

Barbiturates—Extremely potent sedatives that induce sleep.

Cataplexy—When a person suddenly loses muscle tone in his or her arms, legs, face, or neck.

Chronobiology—The study of biological rhythms.

Circadian rhythms—Biological functions that repeat each day at approximately the same time; from the Latin words *circa dia* meaning "about a day."

CPAP (continuous positive airway pressure) device—A mask worn over the nose during sleep that constantly and gently pumps air through the nasal passages to prevent sleep apnea.

Electroencephalograph (EEG)—A device for measuring brain waves.

Half-life—The length of time it takes for the body to metabolize or eliminate half of a drug taken.

Hypnagogic hallucinations—Bizarre and often frightening dreams and sounds that occur during the onset or waking up from cataplexy.

Hypothalamus—A region in the brain that controls sleep and biological rhythms.

Insomnia—Difficulty falling asleep or getting back to sleep after waking during the night.

Jet lag—A temporary maladaptation of the brain and body's biological rhythms when we travel to a new time zone.

Limbic system—Brain regions involved in controlling emotions.

Medulla—Area of the brain stem involved in generating sleep and orchestrating the cycling between the various stages of non-REM sleep, REM sleep, and waking.

Melatonin—A hormone produced by the brain's pineal gland and thought to promote sleep.

Narcolepsy—A complex sleep disorder in which the person repeatedly feels an intense urge to fall asleep at many times throughout the day.

Neuron—Nerve cell in the brain.

Neurotransmitters—Chemical messengers in the brain. Common neurotransmitters include serotonin, glutamate, dopamine, gamma aminobutyric acid (GABA), noradrenaline, and histamine.

Nightmares—Vivid dreams with disturbing content that often cause the person to wake up.

Non-REM sleep—Sometimes called "quiet sleep," it occurs in four stages of gradually deepening rest.

Over-the-counter (OTC) medication—Any medication you can buy at your local pharmacy or grocery store without a prescription.

Periodic limb movements in sleep (PLMS)—A sleep disorder in which people move their limbs (particularly the legs) during sleep.

Pons—Area of the brain stem involved in generating sleep and orchestrating the cycling between the various stages of non-REM sleep, REM sleep, and waking.

Rapid eye movement (REM) sleep—A state of consciousness when most dreaming occurs, characterized by rapid movements of the eyes back and forth; also called "active sleep."

REM behavior disorder (RBD)—In this sleep disorder, when the brain enters REM sleep, it does not send the proper signal to the skeletal muscles to temporarily paralyze you while you dream. The result is that people actually act out portions of their dream or the entire dream.

Restless legs syndrome (RLS)—A sleep disorder in which a person feels an irresistible urge to move his or her legs to alleviate creeping, tingling, cramping, or painful feelings in the legs.

Serotonin—A neurotransmitter thought to be involved in regulating sleep, anxiety, mood, and various aspects of behavior.

Sleep apnea—A breathing disorder characterized by brief interruptions of breathing during sleep.

Sleep bruxism—A fairly common sleep disturbance characterized by clenching of the jaw and/or grinding of the teeth during sleep without the person's awareness.

Glossary

Sleep-related eating disorder—A kind of sleepwalking where the person gets up (after falling asleep), goes to the kitchen, and proceeds to eat a substantial amount of food, then returns to bed and awakens the next morning with no memory of it.

Sleeptalking—Also called somniloquy, this sleep disorder is characterized by either nonsense babbling or mumbling a few words, and at times the person can utter complete coherent sentences. Sleeptalking usually occurs in Stages 1 or 2 of non-REM sleep.

Sleep terrors—A sleep disturbance in which the person appears to wake up screaming and terrified and may cry inconsolably for several minutes. Although the person is not fully awake, the sufferer often shows several physical signs of fear, such as sweating, dilated pupils, and increased blood pressure. Also called night terrors.

Sleepwalking—Also called somnambulism, this sleep disturbance is when a person typically sits up and gets out of bed and moves around the room with clumsy or purposeless movements. These episodes can last from 15 seconds to 30 minutes and usually occur during the first episode of Stage 4 non-REM sleep.

Thalamus—A region in the brain that serves as a relay station for nerve signals from the brain stem to the cortex.

Notes

1 Eric H. Chudler, Ph.D. "How Much Do Animals Sleep?" Available online at http://faculty.washington.edu/chudler/chasleep.html.

2 H. P. Roffwarg, J. N. Muzio, and W. C. Dement, "Ontogenetic Development of the Human Sleep-dream Cycle," *Science* 152 (1996): 604–619.

3 *National Sleep Foundation.* Available online at http://www.sleepfoundation.org.

4 *National Sleep Foundation.* Available online at http://www.sleepfoundation.org.

5 R. Debon, E. Boselli, R. Guyot, et al., "Chronopharmacology of Intrathecal Sufentanil for Labor Analgesia: Daily Variations in Duration of Action," *Anesthesiology* 101 (2004): 978–982.

6 L. W. Foderaro, "Whose Fault is It When the Medicated Run Amok?" *New York Times* (October 28, 1994): A29.

7 S. E. McCabe, J. R. Knight, C. J. Teter, H. Wechsler, "Non-medical Use of Prescription Stimulants Among U.S. College Students: Prevalence and Correlates from a National Survey," *Addiction* 100 (2005): 96–106.

8 C. Poulin, "Medical and Nonmedical Stimulant Use Among Adolescents: From Sanctioned to Unsanctioned Use," *Canadian Medical Association Journal* 165(2001): 1039–1044.

9 *National Sleep Foundation.* Available online at http://www.sleepfoundation.org.

Bibliography

"Bedtime Routine and Sleep Hygiene." *Sleep-Deprivation.com*. Available online at http://www.sleep-deprivation.com/html/sleep-basics.php3.

"Caffeine Content of Beverages, Foods and Drugs." *Holy Mountain Trading Company*. Available online at http://www.holymtn.com/tea/caffeine_content.htm.

Cardinal, Florence. "Sleep Disorders." *About.com*. Available online at http://sleepdisorders.about.com.

"College Sleep Deprivation." *Sleep Disorder Channel*. Available online at http://www.sleepdisorderchannel.net.

"Ephedra Side Effects." *Ephedrine News*. Available online at http://www.ephedrine-news.com.

Hobson, J. A. *Sleep*. New York: Scientific American Library, 1989.

"Insomnia, Sleep Aids, and Stimulant Products." *MedicineNet.com*. Available online at http://www.medicinenet.com/sleep_aids_and_stimulants/article.htm.

Kryger, M., T. Roth, and W. C. Dement. *Principles and Practice of Sleep Medicine*, 2nd edition. Philadelphia: W. B. Saunders, 1994.

National Sleep Foundation. Available online at http://www.sleepfoundation.org.

Office of Communications and Public Liaison, National Institute of Neurological Disorders and Stroke. "Brain Basics: Understanding Sleep." *National Institute of Neurological Disorders and Stroke*. Available online at http://www.ninds.nih.gov/disorders/brain_basics/understanding_sleep_brain_basic.htm.

"Overview of Sleep Disorders." *Talk About Sleep*. Available online at http://www.talkaboutsleep.com/sleep-disorders.

Richards, David W. "Night Terrors." *Night Terror Resource Center*. Available online at http://www.nightterrors.org.

Sack, R. L., A. J. Lewy, M. Rittenbaum, and R. J. Hughes. "Chronobiology and melatonin." In: *Psychoneuroendocrinology—The Scientific Basis of Clinical Practice*. Washington, DC: American Psychiatric Publishing, 2003, pp. 83–105.

"Sleep Aids." *Merck.com*. Available online at http://www.merck.com/mmhe/sec02/ch018/ch018i.html.

"Sleep Basics." *Talk About Sleep*. Available online at http://www.talkabout-sleep.com/sleepbasics/sleepbasics.htm.

"Sleep Disorders." *Neurology Channel*. Available online at http://www.neurologychannel.com/sleepdisorders.

Sleepnet.com. Available online at http://www.sleepnet.com.

WebSciences International and Sleep Research Society. "Basics of Sleep Behavior." Available online at http://www.sleephomepages.org/sleepsyllabus/sleephome.html.

"What Are Stimulants?" *Drug-addiction.com*. Available online at http://www.drug-addiction.com/stimulants.htm.

Further Reading and Websites

FURTHER READING

Dement, W. C., and C. Vaughan. *The Promise of Sleep.* New York: Dell, 2000.

Hauri, P., and S. Linde. *No More Sleepless Nights.* New York: John Wiley, 1996.

WEBSITES

http://www.sleepfoundation.org
National Sleep Foundation

www.nightterrors.org
Night Terror Resource Center

http://www.sleepnet.com
Sleepnet.com

http://www.sleepfoundation.org
Sleep and Health

http://www.sleep-deprivation.com
Sleep-Deprivation.com

http://www.sleepdisorderchannel.net
Sleep Disorder Channel

http://www.talkaboutsleep.com
Talk About Sleep

http://www.sleephomepages.org
WebSciences International and Sleep and Research Society

Index

Index

Picture Credits

Credits

Excedrin is a registered trademark of Bristol-Myers Squibb Company; Excedrin P.M. is a registered trademark of E.R. Squibb & Sons LLC.; Gabitril is a registered trademark of Cephalon, Inc.; Geodon is a registered trademark of Pfizer Inc.; Gin Zing is a trademark of Walgreen Company Corp.; Good Night's Sleep is a registered trademark of Med Gen Inc.; Halcion is a registered trademark of Pharmacia &Upjohn Company, LLC.; Haldol is a registered trademark of Johnson & Johnson Corp.; Imovane is a registered trademark of Aventis Pharma S.A. Corp.; Inderal is a registered trademark of Wyeth Corp.;

Klonopin is a registered trademark of Hoffmann-La Roche Inc.; Lamictal is a registered trademark of Burroughs Wellcome Co. Corp.; Lunesta is a registered trademark of Sepracor Inc.; Luvox is a registered trademark of Solvay Pharma Properties, Inc.; Mellodyn is a registered trademark of BioNeurix Corp.; Metabolife is a registered trademark of Metabolife International, Inc.; Metabolift is a registered trademark of ISI Brands Inc.; Midol is a registered trademark of Bayer Corporation; Mini Thin is a registered trademark of Body Dynamics, Inc.; Nembutal is a registered trademark of Abbott Laboratories Corp.; Neurontin is a registered trademark of Warner-Lambert Company LLC. Nodoz is a registered trademark of E.R. Squibb & Sons LLC.; Norpramin is a registered trademark of Merrell Pharmaceuticals Inc.; Nyquil is a registered trademark of Richardson-Vicks Inc.; Nytol is a registered trademark of Block Drug Company, Inc.; Paxil is a registered trademark of Smithkline Beecham Corporation; ProSom is a registered trademark of Abbott Laboratories Corp.; ProVigil is a registered trademark of Genelco S.A. Joint Stock Company; Prozac is a registered trademark of Eli Lilly and Company Corporation;

Quick Lift is a registered trademark of 206 Macopin Corp.; Red Bull is a registered trademark of Red Bull GmbH LLC.; Restoril is a registered trademark of Novartis Pharmaceuticals Corp.; Ripped Fuel is a registered trademark of ISI Brands Inc.; Risperdal is a registered trademark of Johnson & Johnson Corp.; Ritalin is a registered trademark of Novartis Corp.; Seconal is a registered trademark of Ranbaxy Pharmaceuticals Inc.; Sectral is a registered trademark of Rhone-Poulenc Rorer S.A. Corp.; Seroquel is a registered trademark of Zeneca Limited LLC.; Simply Sleep is a registered trademark of Johnson & Johnson Corp.; Sleep-Eze is a registered trademark of Medtech Products, Inc.; Sleepinal is a registered trademark of Blairex Laboratories, Inc.; Sleep-Max is a registered trademark of Vitamin Classics, Inc.; Sominex is a registered trademark of Smithkline Beecham Corp; Somnitrol is a registered trademark of Rob Dente; Somnulin is a registered trademark of Rob Dente; Sonata is a registered trademark of King Pharmaceuticals Research And Development, Inc.; Sound Sleep is a registered trademark of Sound Sleep LLC.; Starbucks is a registered trademark of Starbucks U.S. Brands LLC.; Stimerall is a registered trademark of 206 Macopin Corp.; Sudafed is a registered trademark of Warner-Lambert Company Corp.;

Tegretol is a registered trademark of Geigy Chemical Corp.; Tenormin is a registered trademark of Zeneca Limited LLC.; Tofranil is a registered trademark of the Novartis Corp.; Topamax is a registered trademark of Johnson & Johnson Corp.; Triaminicin is a registered trademark of Novartis AG Corp.; Tylenol is a registered trademark of The Tylenol Company; Tylenol P.M. is a registered trademark of The Tylenol Company; Unisom is a registered trademark of Pfizer Inc.; Unisom Sleepgels is a registered trademark of Pfizer Inc.; Valium is a registered trademark of Roche Products Inc.; Versed is a registered trademark of Hoffmann-La Roche Inc.; Visken is a registered trademark of Novartis AG Corp.; Vivactil is a registered trademark of Pliva, Inc.; Vivarin is a registered trademark of Smithkline Beecham Corp.; Xenadrine is a registered trademark of Cytodyne LLC; Xyrem is a registered trademark of Orhan Medical, Inc.; Zoloft is a registered trademark of Pfizer Inc.; Zyprexa is a registered trademark of Eli Lilly and Company Corp.; Zyrtec is a registered trademark of Societe Anonyme Corp.;

About the Author

M. Foster Olive received his Bachelor's degree in Psychology from the University of California at San Diego and his Ph.D. in neuroscience from the University of California at Los Angeles. He is currently an Assistant Professor in the Center for Drug and Alcohol Programs at the Medical University of South Carolina. His research focuses on the neurobiology of addiction, and he has been published in numerous academic journals, including *Psychopharmacology* and *The Journal of Neuroscience.*

About the Editor

David J. Triggle is a University Professor and a Distinguished Professor in the School of Pharmacy and Pharmaceutical Sciences at the State University of New York at Buffalo. He studied in the United Kingdom and earned his B.S. degree in Chemistry from the University of Southampton and a Ph.D. degree in Chemistry at the University of Hull. Following post-doctoral work at the University of Ottawa in Canada and the University of London in the United Kingdom, he assumed a position at the School of Pharmacy at Buffalo. He served as Chairman of the Department of Biochemical Pharmacology from 1971 to 1985 and as Dean of the School of Pharmacy from 1985 to 1995. From 1995 to 2001 he served as the Dean of the Graduate School, and as the University Provost from 2000 to 2001. He is the author of several books dealing with the chemical pharmacology of the autonomic nervous system and drug-receptor interactions, some 400 scientific publications, and has delivered over 1,000 lectures worldwide on his research.